THE COMPLETE

FOOD SOLUTION

For INFLAMMATION & AUTOIMMUNE DISEASES

100+ Natural Recipes and Ingredients for Flare up Management

TABLE OF CONTENT

INTRODUCTION

Developed countries including the US, UK, Canada, and Australia are seeing an alarming increase in cases of chronic inflammation and autoimmune illnesses. More than 23.5 million individuals in the US are believed to be affected by autoimmune illnesses, as reported by the NIH. A similar proportion of the population in the United Kingdom deals with an autoimmune disorder. Autoimmune disorders, including lupus, rheumatoid arthritis, type 1 diabetes, and type 2 diabetes, have also been on the rise in Australia and Canada.

According to research, autoimmune illnesses are now more widespread than cancer and rank among the top health problems globally. Beyond the conventional autoimmune spectrum, chronic inflammation has been associated with a broad variety of health problems, including obesity, diabetes, cancer, heart disease, and inflammation, the body's normal reaction to injury and infection.

Some of the most prominent elements of modern lifestyles that are thought to aggravate inflammation are food, stress, pollution, and lack of physical activity. The prevalence of processed foods in these nations, which are rich in sugar and refined carbohydrates, increases the risk of inflammation-related diseases among the population. A growing number of individuals are turning to dietary and lifestyle modifications as a means of controlling or avoiding inflammatory and autoimmune disorders.

Knowing How Food, Inflammation, and Autoimmune Health Are Related

One of the simplest and most accessible ways to change inflammation and autoimmune health is via diet. In addition to providing nourishment, food affects the body's response to stressors and potential threats.

The foods we choose to eat may either promote healing or exacerbate chronic inflammation. For example, meals high in omega-6 fatty acids, which are included in many processed foods, might exacerbate inflammation, while a diet high in omega-3 fatty acids, which are present in foods like walnuts and salmon, may help reduce it. A closer look at how several foods affect inflammation is provided below:

- Processed meals and sweets: Highly processed meals are often high in sugar, refined carbohydrates, and unhealthy fats that may cause insulin and blood sugar imbalances, which over time can cause inflammation.
- Dairy and Gluten: These are common allergens and may cause inflammation, especially in sensitive people. Dairy and gluten may cause immunological responses in people with autoimmune diseases, which might make symptoms worse.
- Omega-3 vs. Omega-6 Balance: These fats must be in a balanced ratio. While omega-6s, which are included in vegetable oils and fried foods, may be pro-inflammatory when out of balance, omega-3s, which are found in foods like walnuts, flaxseeds, and fatty fish, are anti-inflammatory.

- Antioxidant-Rich Foods: Antioxidant-rich foods, such leafy greens, almonds, and berries, fight oxidative stress, which may lead to chronic inflammation.
- Herbs and Spices: Garlic, ginger, and turmeric are among the ingredients that naturally reduce inflammation. These might be important dietary supplements for lowering inflammation.

Finding dietary triggers is very important for those with autoimmune diseases. In autoimmune illnesses, the immune system mistakenly attacks healthy cells, causing tissue damage and inflammation. Inflammatory foods may exacerbate these immune responses, aggravating symptoms and perhaps causing more frequent or severe flare-ups.

Do Flare-Ups Exist? Identifying and Minimizing Triggers

A "flare-up" is a period of time when symptoms of autoimmune and inflammatory diseases suddenly become more severe. A number of factors, including stress, sleep deprivation, changes in the environment, and—most importantly—food, may cause flare-ups. Here's a closer look at the factors that lead to flare-ups and how dietary changes may help reduce their frequency:

The following are the main causes of flare-ups:

- Dietary Choices: Foods such as gluten, dairy, sugar, and alcohol are key offenders. Meals that are highly processed and include chemicals or preservatives may also cause the body to respond inflammatorily.
- Stress: Hormonal imbalances brought on by high stress levels may make the immune system more prone to overreaction.
- Environmental Factors: Inflammatory pathways may be triggered by exposure to pollutants or certain substances, especially in those with autoimmune sensitivity.
- Sleep and Exercise: Since they impede the body's natural healing processes, poor sleep and inactivity may increase inflammation.

Identifying the Initial Indications of a Flare-Up:

Being aware of the early warning signs of a flare-up might help you avoid one. Increased joint pain, fatigue, gastrointestinal issues, skin sensitivity, and mental changes are typical signs. People may better identify their specific triggers by monitoring these symptoms in relation to dietary and lifestyle changes.

By gradually reintroducing foods and monitoring reactions, **elimination diets** (like the Autoimmune Protocol, or AIP) may be able to assist pinpoint specific dietary triggers. Over time, many find that adhering to an anti-inflammatory, whole-food diet reduces the frequency and intensity of flare-ups.

How This Book Can Help: A Handbook on Using Food to Heal

This book aims to serve as a useful manual for anybody looking to use food to reduce inflammation and manage autoimmune diseases. We will discuss:

- Scientific Insights: An approachable overview of the science behind autoimmune disorders and inflammation that explains why some foods may have a greater impact on you than others.
- The carefully crafted meal plans and more than 100 recipes in this section are designed to reduce inflammatory triggers, increase healing nutrients, and give you more control over your health
- Nutritional Strategies: We will examine nutritional approaches, including elimination diets, the Mediterranean diet, and the anti-inflammatory diet, and provide guidance on how to apply these practices in a sustainable way.
- Practical Tools: To assist you successfully follow an anti-inflammatory diet, we'll provide tips on grocery shopping, label reading, and food preparation in addition to recipes.
- Lifestyle advice: We provide a comprehensive strategy to reduce inflammation that goes beyond diet alone, including suggestions for improving sleep quality, stress management techniques, and moderate exercise.

This book encourages you to take charge of your health journey by offering a methodical approach that will help you make informed choices. You'll gain confidence in your capacity to manage symptoms, prevent flare-ups, and adopt a healthy lifestyle that supports long-term wellness with simple-to-follow guidelines on foods that are good for inflammation.

PART 1: The Foundation of Anti Inflammatory Eating

Anyone going through the complicated terrain of inflammation and autoimmune health must comprehend the fundamentals of anti-inflammatory nutrition. Knowing what inflammation is, why it happens, and how it may both benefit and hurt our bodies is the first step on this journey. This fundamental understanding helps in illuminating the potent role that nutrition has in reducing inflammation, which may have a substantial effect on autoimmune health.

The Study of Autoimmune Diseases and Inflammation

The human body has an amazing defensive mechanism that keeps people healthy, fights off diseases, and heals wounds. One important aspect of this process is inflammation. But prolonged or misdirected inflammation may cause long-term health problems, especially for those with autoimmune illnesses.

Inflammation Causes?

The body's natural reaction to damage or illness is inflammation. Consider it the body's emergency reaction mechanism. For instance, when you cut your finger, the surrounding tissue swells, becomes heated, and turns red. This is inflammation in action, an immunological reaction in which your body releases white blood cells to heal damaged tissues and fend against dangerous intruders.

Chronic (long-term) inflammation is a separate matter, even if acute (short-term) inflammation is advantageous and required for healing. Chronic inflammation, which often arises from the immune system being in a "fight" state for longer than necessary, may linger for months or even years. Chronic inflammation may be detrimental and broad, causing persistent damage to organs and tissues, in contrast to acute inflammation, which is confined and goes away after healing.

Chronic inflammation may be caused by a number of factors:

- Improper Diet: Inflammation may be exacerbated by diets high in processed foods, sweets, bad fats, and additives. These foods alter insulin levels and cause the body to generate inflammatory markers.
- Environmental Toxins: Prolonged inflammatory reactions may result from immune system stress caused by pollution, chemicals, and exposure to toxins.

- Chronic Stress: Prolonged stress raises the production of cortisol, which over time may impair immunity and fuel inflammation.
- A sedentary lifestyle may exacerbate inflammation because it impairs circulation, which is necessary to eliminate inflammatory substances.
- Infections: Chronic inflammation may result from bacterial or viral infections that persist because the body keeps producing an immune response long after the illness should have subsided.

Autoimmune disorders cause persistent inflammation and damage because the immune system erroneously attacks healthy tissues as if they were dangerous intruders. By identifying the underlying causes of inflammation, we may better manage it with dietary and lifestyle modifications, which we'll discuss throughout this book.

Typical Autoimmune Conditions and Their Signs

When the body's immune system targets its own cells, autoimmune disorders result. Each of the more than 80 known autoimmune diseases has a distinct set of symptoms. Although any region of the body might be impacted by these illnesses, certain symptoms and ailments are more prevalent than others. An outline of some of the most common autoimmune diseases is provided below:

1. RA, or rheumatoid arthritis

Causes discomfort, swelling, and stiffness in the joints, especially the hands and feet.
Joint discomfort, exhaustion, fever, and loss of joint function are some of the symptoms. The skin, eyes, lungs, and heart may all be impacted by RA.
Triggers: Processed foods and high sugar are known to exacerbate inflammation in RA patients.

2. The second is lupus

(Also known as systemic lupus erythematosus, or SLE) Systemic lupus erythematosus, or SLE.
Fatigue, joint discomfort, rash, fever, and inflammation of the organs are some of the symptoms. A "butterfly" face rash is common.
Triggers: Sunlight exposure, stress, and certain foods may all cause symptoms of lupus.

3. Diabetes Type 1

This kind of diabetes is characterized by elevated blood sugar levels brought on by the immune system attacking the pancreatic cells that produce insulin.
Increased thirst, frequent urination, exhaustion, and impaired vision are some of the symptoms.
Triggers: Although diet does not directly cause type 1 diabetes, several foods may affect inflammation and blood sugar regulation.

4. MS, or multiple sclerosis

Multiple sclerosis is a neurological disorder in which the immune system targets the sheath that surrounds nerve fibers, causing problems with brain-body communication.
Symptoms: Vision difficulties, balance problems, numbness, and muscle weakness.
Triggers: For some people, stress and certain foods, such as dairy and gluten, may exacerbate MS symptoms.

5. Psoriasis

A skin disorder in which skin cells accumulate quickly, resulting in dry, itchy areas and scales.
Symptoms: Itching, soreness, dry and cracked skin, and red spots with silvery scales.
Triggers: Stress, processed foods, and alcohol are often cited as psoriasis triggers.

Although the symptoms and dietary needs of each autoimmune illness are different, one thing is always the same: lowering inflammation via food may help people with these disorders manage their symptoms and live better lives

Key Nutritional Deficiencies in Autoimmune Conditions

People with autoimmune diseases may have worsening symptoms due to nutritional deficits. It is even more crucial for people with autoimmune illnesses to acquire the nutrients they need since inflammation may make it more difficult for the body to absorb nutrients. Some of the most prevalent dietary deficits in people with autoimmune diseases are listed below:

1. Vitamin D: Essential for bone health, inflammatory management, and immunological modulation.
Fatigue, bone discomfort, muscular weakness, and an increased risk of infection are all symptoms of a deficiency.
   - Sources: Fortified meals, fatty fish (such salmon and mackerel), and sun exposure.

2. Fatty Acids Omega-3: Omega-3 fatty acids, which are well-known for their anti-inflammatory qualities, aid in the regulation of inflammation and promote brain health.
Joint discomfort, brittle nails, dry skin, and elevated inflammation are all signs of a deficiency.
   - Sources: Walnuts, flaxseeds, chia seeds, and fatty fish (trout, sardines, and salmon).

3. Magnesium: Vital for blood pressure control, muscular health, and nerve function. Magnesium also aids with inflammation reduction.
   - Deficiency Symptoms: heart palpitations, mood swings, fatigue, and cramping in the muscles.
   - Sources: Dark chocolate, whole grains, seeds, nuts (almonds, cashews), and leafy greens.

4. Vitamin B12: Essential for DNA synthesis, red blood cell creation, and neurological health.
Deficiency symptoms include weakness, anemia, fatigue, and cognitive issues.
Meat, dairy products, fortified cereals, and B12 supplements for plant-based diets are some of the sources.

5. Zinc: Vital for anti-inflammatory, wound-healing, and immunological processes.
   - Deficiency Symptoms: Slow wound healing, diarrhea, hair loss, and weakened immunity.
   - Sources: Nuts, seeds, legumes, meat, and seafood.

6. Iron: Vital for energy synthesis, immunological function, and blood oxygen transport.
The symptoms of a deficiency include weakness, fatigue, pale skin, and recurrent infections.

- Sources: Leafy greens, beans, red meat, and fortified cereals.

People with autoimmune diseases may aid their body's healing processes by addressing these important deficiencies via diet, supplements, or both. To successfully manage autoimmune symptoms and reduce inflammation, a well-balanced diet with a range of nutrient-dense foods is essential.

Foods to Steer Clear of: That Increase Inflammation

The foods we eat on a daily basis have a significant impact on whether inflammation in the body is reduced or increased. Certain meals may promote healing and lower inflammation, while others might have the opposite effect. Knowing which foods may be exacerbating symptoms is crucial for those with autoimmune diseases or those controlling inflammation.

Foods Processed and Unknown Additives

Because they are so handy, processed foods are a mainstay of many diets. Nevertheless, these meals often include unidentified substances that might exacerbate inflammation and interfere with the body's normal functions.

1. Gaining Knowledge about Processed Foods

Foods that have undergone changes from their natural condition are referred to as processed foods. This may include everything from packaged snacks, chips, and frozen dinners to things like fast noodles and sugary cereals. Processing often entails adding substances that the body finds difficult to digest or absorb, although it is sometimes done to increase shelf life or make a product more pleasant.

2. Unknown Ingredients in Prepared Foods

Despite their seemingly harmless appearance, many processed foods include substances that may lead to inflammation in the body. Here are some typical additives to be aware of:

To increase the shelf life of processed foods, artificial preservatives such as BHA (butylated hydroxyanisole) and BHT (butylated hydroxytoluene) are added. Although they keep food from spoiling, research indicates that they may cause inflammation in some individuals.

Artificial Colors and Flavors: These are substances that are added to food to improve its flavor and look, but they may cause inflammatory and allergic reactions in those who are sensitive to them.

Monosodium glutamate, or MSG, is a flavor enhancer that is used in a variety of savory meals, including soups and snacks. After taking MSG, some individuals have symptoms including flushing, sweating, and headaches, which are signs of an inflammatory reaction.

Emulsifiers: Often found in items such as baked goods, ice cream, and salad dressings, emulsifiers aid in the blending of components that don't combine naturally. Nevertheless, research indicates that certain emulsifiers may cause inflammation and disturb the gut microbiota.

3. The Inflammatory Effects of Processed Foods

Generally speaking, processed foods are poor in nutrients and high in calories. Frequent use might lead to a persistent low-grade inflammatory condition because the body is deficient in vital vitamins and minerals required for balanced health. Furthermore, the chemicals utilized to prepare food are often foreign to the body, which triggers an immunological reaction since the body perceives them as intruders.

You may lessen your consumption of these inflammatory ingredients by avoiding processed foods as much as you can or by selecting less processed substitutes. The greatest approach to nourishing the body and reducing the effects of hidden additives is to choose complete, natural meals.

Sugar, Refined Carbohydrates, and Inflammatory Fats

Even though a lot of us like fried meals, sweets, and refined carbohydrates, these are some of the worst things for causing inflammation in the body. Here's a deeper look at their role in inflammatory reactions and the reasons an anti-inflammatory diet is the best way to reduce them.

1. Sugar

Consuming sugar causes the release of cytokines, which are indicators of inflammation. The body releases insulin to assist metabolize the sugar when blood sugar levels rise, causing a brief energy boost that is followed by a collapse. The body is stressed by frequent surges and crashes, which eventually lead to inflammation.

Unknown Sugars in Common Foods: Sugar isn't simply found in candies and drinks. Foods like breads, spaghetti sauces, and salad dressings often contain hidden sugars. You may prevent eating more sugar than you think by looking for added sugars on labels.

2. Carbohydrates Refined

Processed grains that have had their fiber, vitamins, and minerals removed are known as refined carbohydrates. White bread, pastries, white rice, and a variety of snack items are a few examples. These meals easily convert to sugar when they lack the fiber and nutrients, which causes blood sugar levels to rise fast.

The Cause of Inflammation by Refined Carbs: Similar to sugar, refined carbohydrates break down quickly, resulting in brief blood sugar rises. Blood sugar swings put the body under stress and may lead to inflammation as the immune system attempts to adjust to the unpredictability. These meals' lack of fiber also makes them less satisfying, which encourages individuals to eat more than they would with whole grains, which exacerbates the issue.

3. Inflammatory Fats

It is well known that certain lipids, particularly trans fats and harmful saturated fats, may lead to inflammation. Particularly dangerous are trans fats, which are artificial fats included in margarine, fast food, and a variety of baked products. When ingested in excess, unhealthy saturated fats—found in fatty meat cuts and full-fat dairy—can also exacerbate inflammation.

The Dangers of Inflammatory Fats: Trans fats and excessive saturated fats cause arterial inflammation and raise the risk of heart disease by boosting "bad" LDL cholesterol levels while decreasing "good" HDL cholesterol. Furthermore, these fats have the ability to cause the body to create pro-inflammatory chemicals, which over time may exacerbate inflammation.

4. Healthy Alternatives

- Natural Sweeteners: Use natural sweeteners, such as honey, maple syrup, or dates, in place of refined sugar. These sweeteners have a lower glycemic index and may lessen blood sugar increases.
- Whole Grains: Whole grains, such as brown rice, quinoa, oats, or whole-grain bread, include fiber that helps control blood sugar levels, so substitute them for refined carbohydrates.
- Healthy Fats: Consume foods high in anti-inflammatory fats, such as almonds, avocados, olive oil, and fatty fish (like salmon), since they may help regulate inflammation in the body.

Dairy, Gluten, and Other Typical Triggers

Although dairy and gluten don't cause inflammation in everyone, they may be frequent triggers for persons with sensitivities, particularly those who have autoimmune diseases. Here are some reasons they may create problems and, if necessary, advice on how to prevent them.

First, gluten: Rye, barley, and wheat all contain the protein gluten. Because it gives dough its elasticity, it's a popular component in bread, pasta, and a lot other processed meals.

Gluten causes an autoimmune reaction that destroys the small intestine in those with celiac disease. Gluten may sometimes result in joint pain, exhaustion, and digestive problems, even in those without celiac disease. These symptoms point to an inflammatory reaction. For those who are sensitive to or intolerant to gluten, this is particularly true.

Substitutes for Gluten-Containing Foods: If gluten exacerbates your symptoms, there are several substitutes, including gluten-free flours (like almond, coconut, and oat flour) and gluten-free grains (such rice, quinoa, and millet).

2. Dairy: Some individuals have trouble digesting the carbohydrates (lactose) and proteins (casein and whey) found in dairy products. For example, bloating, gas, and discomfort are symptoms of an inflammatory response

in the stomach that may be brought on by lactose intolerance. For some, casein may function as an allergen, causing an immunological reaction that exacerbates inflammation.

Skin conditions like hives, eczema, or acne, as well as digestive disorders, might be signs of dairy sensitivity. Dairy avoidance may help persons with autoimmune disorders have less symptoms.

Dairy-Free Alternatives: Almond milk, coconut milk, and oat milk are just a few of the many dairy-free options that are available. These substitutes are also often used to make dairy-free cheeses, yogurts, and ice creams.

The third common trigger is soy. While it may be a good source of protein, some individuals are sensitive to it. Try staying away from soy and selecting substitutes like quinoa, lentils, or chickpeas if it appears to exacerbate your symptoms.

Nightshade Vegetables: Potatoes, eggplants, tomatoes, and peppers are examples of nightshades. For many, they are nourishing, but for others with autoimmune diseases, they worsen inflammation or joint discomfort.

Alcohol: Excessive alcohol use might aggravate the gastrointestinal tract and increase inflammation. Moderation is essential, and if someone notices that alcohol exacerbates their symptoms, it may be helpful for them to abstain from it completely.

Foods for Healing: Ingredients and Nutrients That Lower Inflammation

Making the switch to an anti-inflammatory diet entails restorative foods that boost the body's defenses, lower inflammation, and alleviate autoimmune and inflammatory disease symptoms. These foods are a vital component of any anti-inflammatory diet since they actively fight inflammation at the cellular level in addition to being nutrient-dense.

Phytonutrients, Omega-3s, and Antioxidants

These three groups—antioxidants, phytonutrients, and omega-3s—all have distinct and complementary functions in reducing inflammation, bolstering the immune system, and advancing long-term health.

1. Fatty Acids Omega-3

Because they are important fats, we must get omega-3 fatty acids from our diet because our bodies are unable to manufacture them on their own. Because of their well-known anti-inflammatory qualities, omega-3 fatty acids are particularly advantageous for those who suffer from autoimmune disorders and chronic inflammation.

Omega-6 fatty acids, which are common in processed foods and may increase inflammation when ingested in excess, are counteracted by omega-3 fatty acids. You may encourage a more healthy inflammatory response and lessen the synthesis of inflammatory chemicals called cytokines by striking a balance between omega-6 and omega-3 fatty acids.

Omega-3 Sources

Fatty fish, such as mackerel, sardines, and salmon, are the finest suppliers of omega-3 fatty acids. Chia seeds, flaxseeds, and walnuts are among plant-based sources of ALA (alpha-linolenic acid), an omega-3 that the body may partly transform into the more powerful EPA and DHA forms that are present in fish. Several times a week, consuming a portion of foods high in omega-3 fatty acids may help reduce inflammation and promote heart and brain function.

The second item is Antioxidants

Free radicals are unstable chemicals that may damage cells and tissues, causing inflammation and an increased risk of chronic illnesses. Antioxidants are substances that shield cells from this damage. Antioxidants prevent cell damage, slow down aging, and promote general health by scavenging free radicals.

Antioxidants lessen oxidative stress, a major cause of inflammation, by stabilizing free radicals. Antioxidants assist maintain a healthy immune response and guard against harm to important organs and tissues by lowering oxidative stress.

Antioxidant Sources

Antioxidants are abundant in fruits and vegetables. Antioxidants are abundant in leafy greens (like spinach and kale), berries (like blueberries, strawberries, and raspberries), and vibrantly colored vegetables (such bell peppers, carrots, and sweet potatoes). Furthermore, dark chocolate and green tea are great antioxidants. Daily consumption of a range of these foods may provide the body a powerful antioxidant boost and aid in the natural reduction of inflammation.

The third is Phytonutrients

Plants contain substances called phytonutrients, also referred to as plant nutrients, which have anti-inflammatory and immune-stimulating qualities. These nutrients may lower the risk of illnesses linked to inflammation and give fruits and vegetables their vivid hues.

Phytonutrients assist the body's natural healing processes and reduce inflammation at the cellular level. They are also associated with enhanced immunity and defense against long-term illnesses including cancer and heart disease.

Phytonutrient Sources

Different kinds of phytonutrients are represented by the colors of fruits and vegetables. For example, lycopene, which has anti-inflammatory properties, is what gives tomatoes and melons their red color. Beta-carotene, which boosts immunity, is abundant in orange foods like sweet potatoes and carrots. Resveratrol, which is found in purple foods like eggplant and grapes, is believed to have heart-healthy properties. You may guarantee a high intake of different phytonutrients that help inflammation reduction by eating a rainbow of colors.

Probiotic-Rich Foods and Digestive Health

Since the digestive tract contains around 70% of the immune system, the stomach is important for controlling inflammation. A balanced immune response depends on a healthy gut, and foods high in probiotics may support the maintenance of a healthy microbiome—the population of good bacteria in the gut.

1. Comprehending the Function of Probiotics in the Gut

Live beneficial bacteria, or probiotics, support intestinal equilibrium. They control the immune system, aid in digestion, and provide defense against dangerous microorganisms. An imbalance in the gut microbiota may worsen autoimmune symptoms and cause inflammation.

2. The Inflammatory-Reduction Effects of Probiotics

By strengthening the gut lining, probiotics help keep dangerous compounds out of the circulation and stop the immune system from reacting. Additionally, they facilitate nutrient absorption and digestion, both of which are critical for controlling inflammation. Furthermore, it has been shown that some probiotic strains directly enhance immune function and lower inflammation.

3. Probiotic Sources

Fermented foods are inherently abundant in live bacteria that promote gut health, making them probiotic-rich diets. Several well-liked options are:

- Yogurt: Has live cultures that promote gut health and digestion. To stay away from extra sugars that might exacerbate inflammation, go for plain, unsweetened yogurt.
- Kefir: A yogurt-like fermented milk beverage that has even more beneficial bacterial strains.
- Sauerkraut: Probiotics and fiber-rich fermented cabbage that promotes intestinal health.
- Kimchi: A classic Korean cuisine with probiotic properties, prepared from fermented veggies and herbs.
- Kombucha: A probiotic and antioxidant-rich fermented tea.
- Miso is a Japanese condiment that is prepared from fermented soybeans and is used in sauces and soups.

Eating a range of foods high in probiotics may help you maintain gut health, which lowers inflammation and boosts immunity.

Natural Anti-Inflammatory Properties of Spices and Herbs

In addition to adding taste to meals, herbs and spices also contain potent molecules that aid in healing and inflammation reduction. For millennia, traditional medicine has used a variety of herbs and spices to reduce inflammation and improve general health.

First, Turmeric:

Curcumin, a substance found in turmeric, has potent anti-inflammatory and antioxidant qualities. Curcumin is a potent natural treatment for inflammatory diseases because it blocks the chemicals that cause inflammation.

You may add turmeric to drinks, soups, and curries. Black pepper includes piperine, a substance that improves the absorption of curcumin, therefore use it with turmeric for optimal absorption.

2. Ginger

Gingerols and shogaols are substances found in ginger that have antioxidant and anti-inflammatory properties. Ginger may help patients with arthritis and other inflammatory disorders feel less pain and inflammation, according to studies

Grated fresh ginger may be used for drinks, stir-fries, and smoothies. Another easy choice is ginger powder, which works well in marinades, oats, and baking.

3. Garlic

Allicin, one of the sulfur compounds found in garlic, has anti-inflammatory properties. Additionally, garlic strengthens the immune system, which aids in the body's better control of inflammation.

Garlic is best enjoyed raw or cooked just a little. To benefit from garlic's anti-inflammatory properties, add minced garlic to marinades, sauces, and dressings.

4. The fourth is Cinnamon

Antioxidants and anti-inflammatory properties found in cinnamon may help lower edema and boost immunity. Additionally, it aids in blood sugar regulation, which indirectly lessens inflammation.

For a warm, spicy taste and added health benefits, add cinnamon to cereal, smoothies, baked goods, and even savory recipes.

Other Helpful Herbs and Spices –

- Rosemary: Has anti-inflammatory properties that promote digestion and cognitive function.
- Oregano: Packed with antioxidants, oregano helps fight off dangerous germs and decrease inflammation.
- Basil: Contains essential oils with anti-inflammatory and antioxidant properties, such as eugenol.

Capsaicin, an ingredient in cayenne pepper, has anti-inflammatory and pain-relieving qualities.

PART 2: Building your Healing Kitchen

Stocking Your Anti-Inflammatory Pantry

Making the shift to a lifestyle that reduces inflammation starts in the kitchen. It's simpler to prepare meals that promote your health, lower inflammation, and provide vital nutrients when you have the correct ingredients on hand.

Having an anti-inflammatory kitchen that is well-stocked doesn't have to be difficult. Investing in wholesome, adaptable foods will position you for success and guarantee that you always have the ingredients on hand to prepare a therapeutic meal.

Crucial Things for Daily Cooking

Complete, nutrient-dense products are essential in an anti-inflammatory kitchen. The following essentials serve as the cornerstone of a healing pantry, enabling you to prepare wholesome, filling meals without depending on processed foods.

1. Healthy Fats and Oils: Reducing inflammation, enhancing cognitive function, and preserving hormonal balance all depend on healthy fats.

- Extra-Virgin Olive Oil: Packed with antioxidants and monounsaturated fats, olive oil is perfect for mild sautéing, salad dressings, and pouring over cooked food.
- Because of its durability, coconut oil is a fantastic option for cooking at high temperatures. Medium-chain triglycerides (MCTs), which are good for the brain, are also found in coconut oil.
- Avocado Oil: Another heart-healthy oil that's great for salad dressings and cooking at high temperatures.
- Omega-3 fatty acids, fiber, and antioxidants are abundant in nuts and seeds, such as flaxseeds, chia seeds, and walnuts. Chia and flax seeds work especially well in smoothies and as a baking egg alternative.

2. Whole Grains: Fiber, which is found in whole grains, assists with digestion, keeps blood sugar levels stable, and lowers the risk of inflammation.

The following are staples to have on hand:

- Quinoa: A complete protein source with a fluffy texture that works well as a basis for stir-fries or in salads.
- Brown Rice: Rich in vitamins and fiber, brown rice complements many different foods and offers a nutty taste.

- Oats: Because of their versatility, oats may be used as a binder in veggie burgers, in baking, or in breakfast bowls. To get the most anti-inflammatory effects, go for steel-cut or old-fashioned oats.

Both millet and buckwheat are gluten-free cereals that provide vital minerals and fiber. Millet may be used as a basis for vegetable bowls, while buckwheat is good for pancakes.

3. Beans and Legumes: Beans and legumes, which are high in fiber, protein, and vital minerals, promote digestive health, which helps control inflammation.
    - Lentils: A flexible choice that cooks rapidly and works well in salads, soups, and stews.
    - Chickpeas: Excellent in salads, hummus, or roasted for a crispy snack.
    - Black Beans and Kidney Beans: Great for stews, chili, and adding protein to other recipes.

4. Spices, Seasonings, and Herbs: Strong anti-inflammatory qualities found in many herbs and spices enhance food's taste and health benefits.
    - Turmeric with Black Pepper: Black pepper increases the absorption of turmeric, which has strong anti-inflammatory properties.
    - Use fresh or powdered ginger to provide warming and anti-inflammatory properties.
    - Cinnamon: Excellent in oatmeal, smoothies, and baked goods; well-known for lowering inflammation and balancing blood sugar.
    - Onion and Garlic Powder: Sulfur chemicals found in garlic help strengthen the immune system, while onion powder adds taste to savory foods.

5. Nuts, Nut Butters, and Seeds: Nuts and seeds, which are rich in fiber, protein, and healthy fats, help keep blood sugar levels steady while lowering inflammation.
    - Almonds, Walnuts, and Cashews: Cashews provide magnesium, which is essential for nerve function, while almonds and walnuts are high in omega-3 fatty acids.
    - Nut butters, such as cashew or almond butter, are excellent for adding to smoothies, spreading over fruits, and mixing into sauces and salads.

Tips for Meal Prep and Batch Cooking on Busy Days

Even on the busiest days, following an anti-inflammatory diet is made simpler with batch cooking and meal preparation. The temptation to go for processed foods is also lessened when meals are prepared ahead of time. To begin, follow these steps:

1. Select Easy Recipes That Keep Well: Certain foods, such as grain bowls, soups, and stews, keep well in the refrigerator or freezer and can become better over time as the flavors combine.
    - Advice: Seek for recipes that are simple to double and call for entire, fresh ingredients. To have wholesome meals available all week, make a big amount on the weekend.

2. Purchasing High-Quality Storage Containers Is Important: Food that is stored properly retains its nutritional content and stays fresh. Because they don't absorb smells and can be safely reheated in an oven or microwave, airtight glass containers are the best option.
    - Advice: For convenience, arrange containers according to meal types (breakfast, lunch, and supper, for example). It's also easier to see what's accessible fast when you use transparent containers.

3. Prep Ingredients Ahead of Time: When preparing meals from scratch, it saves time to prepare components like chopped veggies, cooked grains, and meats in advance.

- Advice: Every week, set aside some time to boil grains, wash and slice veggies, and portion out meats like tofu or chicken. To make assembling salads, stir-fries, or grain bowls easier, keep these items in the refrigerator.

4. Make Use of Freezer-Friendly Recipes: You may prepare meals in advance for hectic weeks without compromising quality by freezing items like soups, casseroles, and pre-marinated meats.

- Advice: Put the name and date of the recipe on freezer bags or containers. Meals that have been refrozen overnight may be reheated and served the following day.

5. Aim for Versatile Ingredients: Ingredients that can be utilized in a variety of dishes, such as baked chicken breast, roasted veggies, or cooked quinoa, save waste and save time.

- Advice: Include adaptable basics that can be quickly turned into a variety of meals by adding different flavors, dressings, or sauces, such as grains, proteins, and greens.

Guides on Selecting High-Quality Grains, Meats, and Produce

Your meals' nutritional content and taste are both influenced by the quality of your components. Here's how you choose the healthiest grains, meats, and vegetables for a diet that reduces inflammation.

1. Produce: The highest concentration of vitamins, minerals, and antioxidants—all crucial for lowering inflammation—can be found in fresh vegetables.

Advice on Choosing Produce:

- Whenever feasible, choose organic products, particularly those on the "Dirty Dozen" list, which are known to have higher levels of pesticide residues
- Choose locally farmed and seasonal vegetables since it is fresher and higher in nutrients.
- Keep an eye out for freshness indicators, such as crisp leaves on greens and no bruising on fruits, as well as bright colors and firm textures.

2. Meats and Seafood: Antibiotics or chemicals found in conventional meats may exacerbate inflammation. Higher amounts of omega-3 fatty acids are among the improved nutritional profiles offered by pasture-raised or grass-fed products

Advice for Choosing Seafood and Meats:

- Select wild-caught seafood, pasture-raised chicken, and grass-fed cattle to get more omega-3 fatty acids and less additives.
- Because toxins may build up in animal fat, choose lean cuts and chop off any visible fat.
- Seek for sustainable seafood sources since they often have less of an effect on the environment and contain fewer toxins.

3. Whole Grains: Fiber, vitamins, and minerals included in whole grains are critical for lowering inflammation and maintaining stable blood sugar levels.

Advice for Choosing Grains:

- To save money and guarantee a consistent supply of basics like brown rice, quinoa, and oats, buy grains in bulk.
- To steer clear of additional sugars or preservatives, read the ingredient list on grains that are packed.
- If you have a gluten sensitivity or believe gluten causes inflammation, choose gluten-free products.

4. Dairy Substitutes: Particularly for those with lactose intolerance or sensitivity, conventional dairy products may sometimes exacerbate inflammation.

Advice on Choosing Dairy Substitutes:

- To stay away from added sugars, look for unsweetened varieties like oat, coconut, or almond milk.
- To make sure you're still receiving vital minerals like calcium and vitamin D, use fortified dairy substitutes.
- Try dairy-free yogurts and cheeses made with cashews or coconut as a foundation; they often have less ingredients than highly processed varieties.

Tools and Techniques for Maximum Nutrient Retention

Choosing the correct foods is just one aspect of eating an anti-inflammatory diet; another is cooking them to optimize their nutritional value. While certain cooking techniques might cause nutritional loss, others can maintain or even increase the nutrients in food.

You may transform your meals into powerful dishes that provide the most anti-inflammatory effects by using these tools and strategies.

Techniques for Cooking That Maintain Nutrients

Nutrients don't have to be sacrificed during cooking. When it comes to maintaining or even increasing the nutritional value of food, some cooking methods are superior to others. Here are a few of the more effective techniques.

- ✓ Steaming: When food is boiled, water-soluble vitamins like vitamin C and B vitamins may be lost; steaming helps preserve these nutrients. It's also among the most delicate cooking techniques, maintaining the food's original taste, texture, and color.
    - ✓ How to use Steam: You may purchase a specialized electric steamer or use a steamer basket over a pot of boiling water. To get veggies like spinach, broccoli, and carrots soft but still crisp, try steaming them for a few minutes.

- ✓ Sautéing and Stir-Frying: Heat-sensitive nutrients like vitamin C and certain antioxidants may be preserved by using quick cooking techniques like sautéing and stir-frying, which need less time and lower heat. The absorption of fat-soluble vitamins (A, D, E, and K) may also be improved by cooking with healthy fat, such as avocado or olive oil.

- ✓ How to Stir-Fry or Sauté: Add your meats or veggies to a skillet with a little oil heated over medium heat. To maintain as much nutritional content as possible while cooking rapidly and evenly, stir regularly.

- Blanching: Blanching is the act of temporarily cooking vegetables in boiling water and then stopping the cooking process by submerging them in freezing water. This method retains nutrients, taste, and color, particularly in veggies that will be frozen or refrigerated.
  - ✓ Methods for Blanching: After adding the veggies to a saucepan of boiling water for one to two minutes, move them to an ice water bath. Broccoli, leafy greens, and green beans all benefit greatly from blanching.

4. Roasting: In addition to enhancing certain antioxidants, such as the carotenoids found in tomatoes and carrots, roasting vegetables brings out their inherent sweetness. Roasting should be done at a moderate temperature to prevent charring, which may produce substances that aren't as healthy.
   - ✓ Methods for Roasting: Spread proteins or vegetables on a baking sheet and preheat the oven to around 375°F (190°C). Roast, turning halfway through, until tender. Add some avocado or olive oil to improve the taste and absorption of nutrients.

5. Cooking under Pressure: Particularly for harder vegetables like potatoes, cereals, and legumes, pressure cooking helps maintain vitamins and minerals by cutting down on cooking time. Additionally, meals cooked under pressure may be simpler to digest.
   - ✓ Using a Pressure Cooker: Because various components need varying cooking times, adhere to the manufacturer's directions. To help the meal cook more rapidly, make sure you use enough water to produce steam.

Methods of Soaking, Sprouting, and Fermentation

Apart from cooking methods, traditional preparation procedures including sprouting, soaking, and fermentation might enhance digestion and boost nutritional availability. These techniques aid in the breakdown of certain dietary ingredients, facilitating the body's absorption of them.

1. Fermentation: Probiotics, or good bacteria, are great for gut health and are encouraged to develop via fermentation. In addition to being high in vitamins B and K2 and enzymes, fermented foods may help balance gut flora, which is important for lowering inflammation.
   - Methods for Home Fermentation: Start with easy dishes like homemade kimchi or sauerkraut. Add salt to the shredded cabbage (or other vegetables) and store in a jar at room temperature. The fermentation process will be initiated by the airborne bacteria, and after a few days, you will have a meal that is high in probiotics.

2. Sprouting: The nutritious content of grains, legumes, nuts, and seeds is increased by sprouting. It decreases substances known as phytates that might obstruct the absorption of minerals and increases the availability of vitamins C and B. Additionally, sprouted foods are simpler to digest, which makes them perfect for those with sensitive stomachs.

- Sprouting Instructions: Soak grains, beans, or seeds overnight after rinsing them. After draining and giving them another washing, place them in a jar with a towel over them to let the air circulate. Rinse them twice a day until sprouts appear (depending on the food, this may take a day or many days). You may consume sprouted foods raw, mildly cooked, or mixed into salads.

3. Soaking: Antinutrients like phytates and lectins, which may obstruct nutrient absorption, are decreased by soaking grains, legumes, and nuts. Additionally, soaking may shorten cooking times and increase digestibility.

- Methods for Soaking: Before cooking, rinse grains and beans after soaking them in water for the whole night. After soaking in water for a few hours, rinse and drain the nuts and seeds. For beans that might upset your stomach if you eat them raw, such as kidney beans, black beans, and chickpeas, soaking is particularly beneficial.

Preparing Meals for Optimal Digestibility

If not cooked carefully, even nutrient-dense meals might be hard to digest. Making sure that food is simple to digest contributes to better nutrient absorption, less inflammation, and less stress on the body. Here's how to make meals that are simple to digest and high in nutrients.

1. Consciously Mix Foods: It might be difficult to digest certain dietary combinations. For instance, different digestive enzymes are needed for starchy carbohydrates and protein-rich meals, which might make it more difficult to break them down simultaneously. Making sensible meal combinations may facilitate better nutrition absorption and digestion.

- How to Mix Foods Together: Think about serving non-starchy veggies with dishes high in protein (e.g., fish with leafy greens). When consuming grains, try to consume them with veggies instead of a lot of protein. Fruit digests rapidly, so it's usually best eaten on its own or as a snack in between meals.

2. Apply Vinegar or Digestive Enzymes: Particularly for those with digestive sensitivity, taking digestive enzymes or adding a dash of apple cider vinegar to meals may aid in food breakdown and enhance digestion.

- How to Utilize Them: Try adding fermented foods like sauerkraut, which naturally includes digestive enzymes, as a condiment to meals, or mix a little apple cider vinegar into a glass of water before meals.

3. Pay Attention to Cooked Foods High in Fiber: Although raw, high-fiber meals may sometimes be difficult for sensitive stomachs to digest, fiber is vital for digestive health and aids in feeding good gut flora. Although they are often simpler to digest than raw meals, lightly cooked foods nevertheless contain fiber.

- How Fiber Can Be Included: For the best gut health, include both soluble and insoluble fiber into your meals. Foods like oats and chia seeds include soluble fiber, which absorbs water and helps create a gel-like material in the stomach that may be calming. Vegetables and whole grains include insoluble fiber, which gives the stool volume and helps avoid constipation.

4. Avoid Cooking Food Too Much or Too Little: Undercooking may make food more difficult to digest, while overcooking might damage nutrients that are sensitive to heat. Achieving the ideal balance guarantees that your meals are nourishing and comfortable on the stomach.

- How to Prepare Food Correctly: Proteins such as meats and eggs should be cooked until they are firm but not rubbery, and vegetables should be cooked lightly until they are soft but still vivid. in order to aid with digestion, ensure grains and legumes are soft enough to chew.

5. Eat with Mindfulness: Chewing triggers digestive enzymes in the mouth, which is where digestion starts. These enzymes may begin breaking down food when you eat consciously and chew your meal properly, which can help with digestion and lessen the likelihood of bloating or discomfort.

- How to Mindfully Eat: Before eating, take a few deep breaths, sit down, and chew every mouthful well. Steer clear of stressful discussions or displays since they might cause your body to shift from "rest and digest" state.

These tools and methods can help you prepare meals that are nutrient-dense, easy on your digestive tract, and anti-inflammatory. By being proficient in these techniques, you may make sure that every meal has the most vitamins, minerals, and other health-promoting substances possible for your body to absorb. You can make the most of every item and produce meals that are both healthful and delectable when your kitchen is ready.

Reading Labels: Steer clear of Unknown Inflammatory Substances

One of the most powerful abilities for anybody wishing to follow an anti-inflammatory diet is knowing how to read product labels. Labels often include substances that seem innocuous but may in fact exacerbate inflammation, making them unclear or deceptive.

Preservatives and additives used in many processed foods are intended to improve texture, taste, or shelf life. Regrettably, several of these compounds have the potential to exacerbate inflammation, particularly in those with autoimmune diseases or compromised immune systems. These are a few of the most prevalent additives to be aware of and the reasons they could be harmful.

- First, let's review what monosodium glutamate (MSG) is. MSG is a flavor enhancer that is often included in canned soups, processed meals, and fast food. For those who are sensitive, MSG may cause responses that include flushing, headaches, and even elevated inflammation. Even though there is conflicting evidence on MSG's effect in inflammation, if you want to lessen possible triggers, it is recommended to stay away from it.
- Aspartame, Sucralose, and Other Artificial Sweeteners: Artificial sweeteners are sugar replacements used in "diet" or "sugar-free" items such as yogurts, candies, and sodas. Artificial sweeteners are low in calories, however they have been linked to increased inflammation and may upset gut flora. It has been shown that aspartame in particular may trigger immunological reactions in certain people.
- Trans Fats: Hydrogenated and Partially Hydrogenated Oils): These are synthetic fats made by solidifying vegetable oils at room temperature with hydrogen. They may be found in baked items, fried dishes, and margarine. Trans fats are a major risk factor for heart disease and are associated with elevated levels of inflammatory markers in the body. Although the FDA has taken action to eliminate trans fats from the food supply, tiny levels may still be present in certain products.
- In order to stop germs from growing and maintain color, processed foods like bacon, hot dogs, and deli meats employ sodium nitrate and sodium nitrite as preservatives. These preservatives may produce substances known as nitrosamines when heated to high temperatures, and these chemicals have been linked to an increased risk of cancer and inflammation.

- High-Fructose Corn Syrup (HFCS): HFCS is a low-cost sweetener derived from corn starch that is included in a variety of processed foods, drinks, and snack foods. Because it is high in sugar, HFCS causes obesity, insulin resistance, and inflammation. Overconsumption of sugar might exacerbate autoimmune disease symptoms.
- Artificial Colors (such as Yellow 5 and Red 40): Synthetic dyes that are used to color beverages, sweets, and processed meals. Artificial coloring has been connected to children's increased hyperactivity and may cause allergic responses. According to some research, they could also make sensitive people more prone to inflammation.
- Carrageenan: a red seaweed-based thickener and stabilizer that is often used in processed meals, dairy products, and plant-based milks. Carrageenan may induce pain and inflammation in the digestive tract, especially in those who have gastrointestinal sensitivities, according to some study.

Comprehending Organic, Non-GMO, and Grass-Fed Labeling Claims

Claims that seem attractive but might be misleading are common on food labels. Let's dissect some of the most prevalent claims you'll come across and explain their true meanings in relation to the anti-inflammatory and food quality advantages.

1. Organic: Genetically modified organisms (GMOs) and synthetic fertilizers, insecticides, and herbicides are not used in the production of organic food. Animals grown without the use of artificial growth hormones or antibiotics are the source of organic animal products. There may be lower pesticide residues and, under some situations, increased antioxidant levels in organic fruit and animal products. Selecting organic products wherever feasible may lessen the strain on your body and maybe minimize inflammation since pesticides can strain the body's detoxification mechanism.
2. The Meaning of Non-GMO: Non-GMO foods are not produced using organisms that have undergone genetic modification. To be sure the product hasn't undergone genetic modification, look for a Non-GMO Project Verified label. Although GMOs are often designed to be resistant to pesticides, they have not been shown to cause inflammation in and of themselves. People with delicate immune systems may benefit from non-GMO foods since they are less likely to contain excessive quantities of pesticides.
3. Grass-Fed: When beef and dairy products are labeled "grass-fed," it indicates that the animals were given a natural diet of grass instead of grain. Antioxidants like vitamin E and omega-3 fatty acids, which reduce inflammation, are more abundant in meats raised on grass. For lowering inflammation, grass-fed beef is a better option than grain-fed meat.
4. Pasture-Raised or Free-Range: Though the quality of their outside time might vary, these expressions typically indicate that animals, like hens, have access to the outdoors. Animal products fed on pasture often have superior nutritious profiles, with greater amounts of vitamin D and omega-3 fatty acids. Since phrases like "free-range" may mean quite different things in different contexts, look for certificates to guarantee quality.
5. Free of Cages: Cage-free eggs may still be housed inside, but the chickens are not housed in tiny cages. Although cage-free eggs may not always have better nutrition, they may be a more moral option if you care about animal welfare. On the other hand, eggs produced on pasture often contain more nutrients.
6. Gluten-Free: Gluten, a protein present in wheat, barley, and rye, is absent from gluten-free meals. For those who have celiac disease or gluten sensitivity, this is crucial. Avoiding gluten helps lessen inflammation in those with autoimmune diseases like celiac disease or gluten sensitivity. But just

because a product is gluten-free doesn't imply it's healthy, so look for sugars and chemicals in processed gluten-free meals.

How to Shop Wisely:

With a few clever suggestions, choosing anti-inflammatory foods at the supermarket may be simple. Here's how to avoid the typical pitfalls of processed meals and position yourself for success.

1. Start by shopping the perimeter: The grocery store's outside boundaries are often where you'll find fresh vegetables, meats, and dairy items. Compared to the boxed and canned products that often include chemicals found in the middle aisles, these foods are typically less processed and higher in nutrients.

- Stock up on fresh produce, lean meats, and healthy foods from the outside aisles to start your shopping journey. Then, only go into the middle aisles for certain products, such as oils, legumes, or whole grains.

2. Pay Close Attention to Ingredient Lists: Examine the contents list to identify any hidden sugars, preservatives, or additions since food packaging may be deceptive.

- Look for products with easily identifiable, brief ingredient lists. A package of nuts, for instance, should ideally just say "nuts" and maybe "salt" and not include any other oils or preservatives.

3. Whenever feasible, choose whole foods: Artificial additives are naturally absent from healthy foods such as lean proteins, whole grains, fresh vegetables, and fruits. They also tend to be lower in calories, sugar, and salt and are full of vital nutrients.

- Choose whole foods over prepackaged ones whenever you can. For instance, buy plain brown rice and season it with your own herbs and spices rather than purchasing a box of seasoned rice.

4. Purchase Basic Ingredients in Bulk: Unprocessed forms of essentials like rice, lentils, nuts, and seeds are often found in bulk bins. These foods are inexpensive and often additive-free.

- Keep supplies of staples like almonds, quinoa, and oats on hand. This is particularly helpful for nuts and seeds, which have anti-inflammatory properties but are often packed with additional sugars or oils.

5. Watch Out for "Health Halos": "Health halos" are statements that make a product seem healthier than it really is, such as "low-fat," "sugar-free," or "high-fiber."

- Examine the nutritional data and ingredients instead of depending only on the promises made on the front of the box. For instance, a "low-fat" yogurt could include a lot of additional sugars to make up for the decreased fat content.

6. Emphasis on Minimally Processed Foods: Inflammatory chemicals, refined oils, and hidden sugars are common in highly processed diets. "Light," "instant," and "microwaveable" foods may have additional additives that lower their nutritional content.

- To do this, choose foods that are as near to their original condition as you can. For instance, choose whole potatoes over boxed mashed potatoes or whole oats over fast oats. This helps you stay away from needless added sugars, oils, and preservatives.

7. Become Informed About Sugar Substitutes and Sweeteners: Hidden sugars or artificial sweeteners like aspartame, sucralose, or high-fructose corn syrup are included in a lot of "health" meals. These may have an adverse effect on gut health and cause inflammation.

- If you need something sweet, look for items that include natural sweeteners. In moderation, maple syrup, honey, or coconut sugar are preferable substitutes. But watch out for hidden sugars in products that are promoted as healthy, including flavored dressings, sauces, and yogurts.

8. Take Care When Purchasing Frozen or Canned Options: Although some canned and frozen meals have additional sugars, salts, or preservatives, frozen fruits and vegetables are often just as nutrient-dense as fresh ones.

- Seek for frozen choices that are labeled "100% vegetables" or "100% fruit" since they don't include any additional additives. Select canned items that have "no salt added" or "in water" as opposed to those that have extra preservatives or sweet syrups.

9. Make Use of Resources and Apps to Make Label Reading Easier: It might be difficult to understand ingredient lists, particularly when the names of the substances are unknown. It is simpler to identify inflammatory substances with the help of certain applications and websites.

- Use applications that assess and score the healthiness of food components, such as Fooducate or EWG's Food Scores. Additionally, they may notify you of possible allergies and other factors that may not be readily apparent on the label.

Gaining the ability to read food labels enables you to steer clear of typical grocery shop traps and make better decisions. You may drastically lower your exposure to hidden inflammatory triggers by recognizing inflammatory components, comprehending the meaning of common labeling claims, and practicing wise shopping.

You can turn every shopping trip into a chance to fill your kitchen with healthy, anti-inflammatory items that really help your health. The basis for eating in a manner that nourishes your body, boosts your immune system, and lowers the risk of inflammation is laid by taking the time to make educated decisions. The foundation for a healthier lifestyle that is simpler to sustain and enjoy over time is laid by this proactive approach to food selection and label reading.

PART 3: The Complete Anti-Inflammatory Meal Plan

AIP Elimination Plan

The Autoimmune Protocol (AIP) Elimination Diet is a science-backed dietary approach specifically designed to help manage autoimmune disease symptoms. By temporarily removing potentially inflammatory foods, it supports the body in reducing systemic inflammation and can help people identify individual dietary triggers that worsen symptoms. The protocol is based on the understanding that certain foods may exacerbate the immune system's attack on healthy tissues in autoimmune conditions, and that removing these foods for a period of time can allow for better control of symptoms and potentially lead to improved long-term health.

Goals of the AIP Elimination Diet

1. Reduce Inflammation: Certain foods can stimulate immune reactions or cause inflammatory responses. Removing these foods helps to reduce the body's inflammatory load, allowing it to focus on healing.

2. Heal the Gut: Research suggests that many individuals with autoimmune diseases have issues with gut health, such as "leaky gut" or intestinal permeability. The AIP diet removes foods that are hard on the gut lining and replaces them with nutrient-dense foods that support gut repair.

3. Identify Triggers: After the elimination phase, foods are reintroduced systematically. This helps people pinpoint specific foods that may worsen symptoms, allowing for a personalized diet that supports their unique needs.

Phases of the AIP Elimination Diet

The AIP diet consists of two main phases:

1. Elimination Phase: All potentially inflammatory foods are removed for a period of time—generally 30 to 90 days, though this can vary. This period allows the body to calm inflammation, reduce symptoms, and reset.

2. Reintroduction Phase: After symptoms improve or stabilize, foods are gradually reintroduced one at a time. This phase is about observing any reactions and determining which foods can be safely incorporated back into the diet without triggering symptoms.

Foods to Avoid During the Elimination Phase

The AIP diet requires the removal of several food categories, which are known to contribute to inflammation or irritation, especially in individuals with autoimmune disorders:

1. Grains: All grains, including wheat, rice, oats, corn, and barley, are eliminated because they can be inflammatory and are common causes of digestive issues.

2. Legumes: Beans, lentils, soy, and peanuts contain compounds that may stimulate the immune system or disrupt gut health.

3. Dairy: Dairy products can be problematic for those with autoimmune conditions, as they may cause inflammation or allergic reactions.

4. Nightshades: Vegetables from the nightshade family (e.g., tomatoes, peppers, potatoes, and eggplants) contain compounds that may irritate the gut and stimulate the immune system in some people.

5. Nuts and Seeds: Though nutrient-dense, nuts and seeds can also be hard on digestion and may trigger immune responses. This includes all nuts, seeds, and seed-based spices (like mustard or cumin).

6. Eggs: While eggs are a healthy food for many people, they contain proteins that some autoimmune individuals find inflammatory.

7. Processed Foods: These often contain additives, preservatives, and artificial ingredients that can lead to inflammation or cause adverse reactions.

8. Added Sugars and Sweeteners: Excess sugar intake has been linked to increased inflammation, so it is best to avoid added sugars and sweeteners like honey, maple syrup, and agave during the elimination phase.

9. Alcohol and Caffeine: Both can be irritating to the gut lining and may exacerbate inflammation.

Foods to Focus On During the Elimination Phase

The focus in the elimination phase is on nutrient-dense foods that support healing, reduce inflammation, and nourish the body. Here are the primary food categories included in the AIP diet:

1. Vegetables (Non-Nightshade): Leafy greens, cruciferous vegetables (like broccoli and cauliflower), and root vegetables (like sweet potatoes and carrots) are nutrient-rich and provide essential vitamins and minerals.

2. Fruits (in moderation): Fruits are generally allowed, though it's advisable to focus on low-glycemic fruits like berries, apples, and pears to avoid blood sugar spikes.

3. Quality Meats and Seafood: Grass-fed, organic meats, and wild-caught fish are encouraged for their high nutrient content, especially omega-3 fatty acids, which are anti-inflammatory.

4. Healthy Fats: Fats from sources like avocados, olives, coconut oil, and fatty fish provide anti-inflammatory omega-3s and other beneficial fats for brain and body health.

5. Herbs and Spices: Fresh herbs (like parsley, rosemary, and cilantro) and certain spices that are not seed-based (like turmeric and ginger) are allowed and provide additional anti-inflammatory properties.

6. Bone Broth: Bone broth is an excellent source of collagen and amino acids, which support gut health and help repair the gut lining.

Reintroduction Phase

Once symptoms have improved and the individual feels stable (often after 30 to 90 days), the reintroduction phase begins. The goal here is to identify specific foods that cause issues, allowing for a customized, long-term diet plan.

How to Reintroduce Foods:

1. Introduce One Food at a Time: Start with the food that is least likely to cause a reaction, such as egg yolks, and then wait for 3–4 days to monitor any symptoms before moving on to the next food.

2. Observe Symptoms: Reactions can manifest immediately or take up to a few days, so it's essential to look for any signs of inflammation, such as joint pain, digestive discomfort, headaches, skin reactions, or fatigue.

3. Track Results: Keeping a food and symptom journal can be helpful to record which foods are tolerated well and which ones should continue to be avoided.

4. Repeat as needed: Continue reintroducing foods gradually and only proceed to the next food if no negative symptoms occur.

Considerations

- Time-Intensive: The diet requires a substantial commitment to meal planning and food preparation, especially during the elimination phase
- Social Limitations: Since the diet restricts many common foods, it may limit dining out or participating in social gatherings centered on food.

30 Days Meal Plan for Autoimmune Conditions

Creating a 4-week Autoimmune Protocol (AIP) meal plan that incorporates both the elimination and reintroduction phases will allow for a careful approach to managing autoimmune symptoms. Here’s how we’ll break it down:

- Weeks 1-3: Strict elimination phase, avoiding common allergens and inflammatory foods, focusing on nutrient-dense, AIP-compliant recipes
- Week 4: Start of the reintroduction phase. We'll introduce one new food every three days to observe any reactions, starting with the least likely to trigger symptoms.

Weeks 1–3: Elimination Phase

Focus entirely on AIP-compliant foods to reset and reduce inflammation. These meals are chosen for their nutrient density, prebiotic qualities, and anti-inflammatory properties.

Week 1
Day 1

- Breakfast: Fermented Beet and Kefir Smoothie (p. 30)
- Lunch: Roasted Fennel & Watercress Salad (p. 98)
- Dinner: Ginger-Turmeric Poached Cod with Wilted Greens (p. 135)
- Side: Green Tea Kombucha-Fermented Radishes (p. 169)
- Snack: Cassava Flour Breakfast Bars (p. 197)

Day 2

- Breakfast: Prebiotic Green Papaya Smoothie (p. 31)
- Lunch: Sea Vegetable & Cucumber Salad (p. 102)
- Dinner: Wild Salmon and Fennel En Papillote (p. 137
- Side: Pickled Watermelon Radish (p. 175)
- Snack: Roasted Carrot and Ginger Energy Balls (p. 202)

...Continue with a variety of AIP-friendly smoothies, soups, and meals as provided.

Week 2

Repeat or rotate the Week 1 meals to avoid new foods but keep things varied.

Week 3

Rotate different meals again from the elimination-phase recipes, focusing on nutrient-dense and anti-inflammatory foods without adding any non-AIP ingredients.

Week 4: Start of Reintroduction Phase

In the reintroduction phase, reintroduce foods in four stages based on their potential inflammatory response. For each food reintroduction, observe for any adverse symptoms over three days before moving on to the next food.

Week 4

Day 1–3: Reintroduce Egg Yolks

- Breakfast: Turmeric-Saffron Omelet with Caramelized Fennel (p. 40) – including egg yolks
- Lunch: Roasted Beet & Microgreens Salad (p. 104)
- Dinner: Mediterranean-Style Mackerel with Herbs (p. 140)
- Side: Braised Artichoke Hearts (p. 193)
- Snack: Cassava Flour Breakfast Bars (p. 197)

Observe for any adverse reactions to egg yolks (digestive issues, skin reactions, etc.). If no reaction, proceed.

Day 4–6: Reintroduce Seed-Based Spices (e.g., cumin, mustard seeds)

- Breakfast: Chicory Root Coffee Smoothie (p. 38)
- Lunch: Roasted Spaghetti Squash (p. 122) – seasoned with seed-based spices
- Dinner: Pan-Seared Halibut with Citrus (p. 145)
- Side: Grilled Japanese Sweet Potatoes with Rosemary (p. 181)
- Snack: Spiced Seed Crackers (p. 212) – includes seed-based spices

Day 7–9: Reintroduce Ghee (clarified butter)

- Breakfast: Golden Milk Scrambled Eggs (p. 45) – with ghee if tolerated
- Lunch: Plantain Tortilla Wraps (p. 112)
- Dinner: Herb-Stuffed Pastured Turkey Breast (p. 149) – cooked in ghee
- Side: Roasted Celeriac with Thyme (p. 183)
- Snack: Golden Turmeric Nut Mix (p. 216)

Day 10–12: Reintroduce White Rice (if well-tolerated on AIP)*

- Breakfast: Moringa Gut-Healing Smoothie (p. 34)
- Lunch: Cassava "Rice" Bowl with Ginger-Glazed Duck (p. 109) – swap with a small portion of white rice
- Dinner: Bone Broth Braised Lamb Shanks (p. 147)
- Side: Kohlrabi Carpaccio (p. 188)
- Snack: Sweet Potato "Toast" Squares (p. 198)

Key Points for Reintroduction

Introduce one new food at a time and observe for 3 days.

- Watch for symptoms like digestive upset, headaches, joint pain, or skin issues.
- If a food triggers symptoms, avoid it and wait until symptoms subside before trying the next.

This phased approach ensures you can accurately identify any triggers and build a sustainable diet around foods that support your health.

PART 4: Recipes for Reducing Inflammation and Managing Autoimmune Flare Ups

Quick Breakfast to Start your Day

Fermented Beet and Kefir Smoothie

(per serving)

Serving Size: 1 smoothie

Calories: 180

Fats: 3g

Carbs: 40g

Protein: 3g

Sugars: 24g (naturally occurring from beets and honey)

Gluten-Free: Yes

Dairy-Free: Yes

Vegan: Yes (if honey is omitted)

1 cup fermented beets (store-bought or homemade)

1 cup coconut kefir (dairy-free)

1 teaspoon fresh ginger, grated

Juice of 1 lime

1 tablespoon honey

1/2 cup coconut water

Put the grated ginger, coconut kefir, lime juice, fermented beets, coconut water, and honey (if using) in a blender.

Blend on high until the mixture is smooth and all the ingredients are properly blended.

If you would like, taste the smoothie and add extra honey to regulate the sweetness.

Transfer the smoothie to a glass and start drinking right away.

Prebiotic Green Papaya Smoothie

(per serving)

Serving Size: 1 smoothie

Calories: 210

Fats: 5g

Carbs: 40g

Protein: 4g

Sugars: 25g (naturally occurring from fruits)

Gluten-Free: Yes

Dairy-Free: Yes

Vegan: Yes

1 cup green papaya, peeled and diced

1/2 cup pineapple, diced

1/2 cup coconut yogurt (dairy-free)

1 teaspoon spirulina powder

1 cup brewed green tea, cooled

Make green tea as directed on the box. Let it cool fully.

Put the chopped green papaya, pineapple, coconut yogurt, spirulina powder, and chilled green tea in a blender.

Process the ingredients on high speed until it becomes creamy and smooth.

If you would like, add extra pineapple or a little bit of honey to the smoothie to change its sweetness.

Transfer the smoothie to a glass and start drinking right away..

Japanese Sweet Potato and Maca Boost

(per serving)

Serving Size: 1 smoothie

Calories: 320

Fats: 7g

Carbs: 60g

Protein: 6g

Sugars: 30g (naturally occurring from sweet potato and dates)

Gluten-Free: Yes

Dairy-Free: Yes

Vegan: Yes

1 medium Japanese purple sweet potato (about 200g), steamed and cooled

1 tablespoon maca powder

1 cup unsweetened almond milk (or other AIP-friendly milk)

1 teaspoon vanilla extract

2 Medjool dates, pitted

The Japanese purple sweet potato should be steamed for 25 to 30 minutes to make it delicate. Peel and cut into bits after letting it cool somewhat.

Put the pitted dates, almond milk, maca powder, boiled sweet potato, and vanilla essence in a blender.

Process the ingredients on high speed until it becomes smooth and creamy.

If additional dates or a little almond milk are needed to thin the mixture, taste it and adjust the sweetness.

Transfer to a dish or glass and start eating right away. You may serve this cold as well.

Cultured Plum and Black Garlic Blend

(per serving)

Serving Size: Approximately 1 cup

Calories: 210

Fats: 3g

Carbohydrates: 49g

Protein: 3g

Sugars: 25g (naturally occurring from plums and honey)

Gluten-Free: Yes

Dairy-Free: Yes

Vegan: Yes (if honey is omitted)

4 black garlic cloves

2 medium purple plums, pitted and chopped

1 cup kombucha (preferably plain or lightly flavored)

2 tablespoons chia seeds

1 tablespoon raw honey (optional)

Put the chia seeds and 1/4 cup of kombucha in a small basin. Soak them for ten to fifteen minutes, or until they expand and take on the consistency of gel.

Put the soaked chia seeds (with any leftover kombucha) and the remainder of the kombucha in a blender along with the chopped purple plums and black garlic.

The next step is to blend the mixture on high until it is smooth. If desired, add raw honey to taste and adjust sweetness.

Transfer the blend into a glass or dish. You may serve it right away or chill it in the refrigerator for a little while..

Moringa Gut-Healing Smoothie

(per serving)

Serving Size: 1 smoothie

Calories: 380

Fats: 17g

Carbs: 48g

Protein: 20g

Sugars: 15g (naturally occurring from banana)

Gluten-Free: Yes

Dairy-Free: Yes

Vegan: No (due to bone broth protein and collagen)

1 teaspoon moringa powder

1/2 cup coconut meat (fresh or frozen)

1 cup bone broth protein (preferably unflavored)

1 ripe banana

1 tablespoon collagen powder

1 cup water or coconut water (for blending)

Scoop out the fresh coconut flesh from the coconut if using. Give it a little time to defrost if using frozen.

Put the banana, collagen powder, bone broth protein, coconut flesh, moringa powder, and water or coconut water in a blender.

Blend on high until the mixture is creamy and all the ingredients are fully blended.

If you would like a thinner consistency, taste the smoothie and add additional water or coconut water.

Transfer to a glass and start drinking right away..

Tiger Nut Horchata Smoothie

(per serving)

Serving Size: 1 smoothie (makes about 2 servings)

Calories: 260

Fats: 9g

Carbs: 45g

Protein: 5g

Sugars: 20g (naturally occurring from dates and tiger nuts)

Gluten-Free: Yes

Dairy-Free: Yes

Vegan: Yes

1 cup soaked tiger nuts (soak in water for at least 12 hours)

2 Medjool dates, pitted

1/2 teaspoon ground cinnamon

1/2 teaspoon vanilla bean paste or 1/2 teaspoon vanilla extract

2 cups filtered water

In case you haven't already, soak the tiger nuts in water for a minimum of 12 hours or overnight. Before usage, drain and rinse.

Put the soaked tiger nuts, powdered cinnamon, pitted Medjool dates, vanilla bean paste, and filtered water in a blender.

Blend for one to two minutes on high, or until the mixture is smooth and creamy. It may be necessary to pause and clean the blender's sides.

To get rid of any solids and achieve a smoother texture, strain the mixture using a fine mesh strainer or a nut milk bag.

Enjoy the horchata smoothie right away after pouring it into glasses, or store it in the fridge for a cool beverage at a later time.

Natto and Berry Probiotic Blast

(per serving)

Serving Size: 1 smoothie

Calories: 250

Fats: 8g

Carbs: 40g

Protein: 10g

Sugars: 15g (naturally occurring from berries)

Gluten-Free: Yes

Dairy-Free: Yes

Vegan: Yes

1/2 cup natto (fermented soybeans, preferably organic)

1 cup mixed berries (such as blueberries, strawberries, and raspberries)

1 tablespoon hemp seeds

1 teaspoon fresh ginger, grated

1 cup coconut water

Rinse the mixed berries and grate the ginger if it hasn't been done before.

Put the natto, grated ginger, hemp seeds, mixed berries, and coconut water in a blender.

Process the ingredients on high speed until it becomes creamy and smooth. If desired, you may need to add more coconut water to change the thickness.

If the combination isn't strictly AIP, add additional berries or a little amount of honey to balance the sweetness.

.

Jerusalem Artichoke Prebiotic Shake

(per serving)

Serving Size: 1 shake

Calories: 350

Fats: 15g

Carbs: 50g

Protein: 8g

Sugars: 25g (naturally occurring from pear and almond butter)

Gluten-Free: Yes

Dairy-Free: Yes

Vegan: Yes (if using plant-based kefir)

1 cup Jerusalem artichoke, peeled and chopped

1 ripe pear, cored and diced

2 tablespoons almond butter (ensure it's AIP-compliant)

1/2 teaspoon ground cinnamon

1 cup coconut kefir or other dairy-free kefir

To prepare the Jerusalem artichoke, boil it in water for ten to fifteen minutes until it is soft. After draining, let cool.

Put the cooked Jerusalem artichokes, peanut butter, ground cinnamon, chopped pear, and coconut kefir in a blender.

Process the ingredients on high speed until it becomes smooth and creamy.

If additional pear or a dash of maple syrup is needed, taste the shake and adjust the sweetness.

Transfer to a glass and start drinking right away. You may also serve this smoothie cold..

Chicory Root Coffee Smoothie

(per serving)

Serving Size: 1 smoothie

Calories: 320

Fats: 12g

Carbs: 58g

Protein: 3g

Sugars: 30g (naturally occurring from banana and dates)

2 tablespoons roasted chicory root (coarsely ground)

1 ripe banana

1 tablespoon raw cacao powder

2 Medjool dates, pitted

1 cup unsweetened coconut milk

Gluten-Free: Yes

Dairy-Free: Yes

Vegan: Yes

To make chicory root coffee, soak chicory root in one cup of boiling water for five to ten minutes. After straining, let it cool a little.

Put the ripe banana, pitted dates, raw cacao powder, coconut milk, and brewed chicory coffee in a blender.

Blend on high until the mixture is smooth and creamy and all the ingredients are properly blended.

If additional dates or a different banana are needed to get the desired sweetness, taste the smoothie and make the required adjustments.

Transfer the smoothie to a glass and start drinking right away..

Dandelion Greens Detox Blend

(per serving)

Serving Size: 1 smoothie (approximately 2 cups)

Calories: 80

Fats: 1g

Carbs: 20g

Protein: 2g

Sugars: 10g (naturally occurring from apple and coconut water)

2 cups fresh dandelion greens, washed and chopped

1 green apple, cored and diced

1/2 cucumber, peeled and diced

1/4 cup fresh mint leaves

1 cup coconut water

Gluten-Free: Yes

Dairy-Free: Yes

Vegan: Yes

Rinse the mint leaves, core and chop the green apple, peel and cut the cucumber, and wash and chop the dandelion greens.

Put the green apple, cucumber, mint leaves, coconut water, and dandelion greens in a blender.

Blend on high until smooth and well mixed. You may add extra coconut water if you desire a thinner consistency.

Transfer to a glass and start drinking right away. You may serve this combination over ice as well.

Turmeric-Saffron Omelet with Caramelized Fennel

(per serving)

Serving Size: 1 omelet

Calories: 320

Fats: 25g

Carbs: 10g

Protein: 18g

Sugars: 3g

Gluten-Free: Yes

Dairy-Free: Yes

Vegan: No (contains eggs)

3 large eggs

1/4 teaspoon saffron threads

1/2 teaspoon turmeric powder

1 medium fennel bulb, sliced thinly

1 tablespoon olive oil (or AIP-friendly fat)

Salt, to taste (optional for AIP)

Fresh herbs (e.g. parsley or chives), chopped, for garnish

Water (for saffron infusion)

To release the taste and color of the saffron threads, soak them in 1 tablespoon of warm water in a small basin for about 10 minutes.

Heat olive oil in a pan over medium heat. Add the sliced fennel and simmer for 10 to 15 minutes, stirring regularly, until it is tender and caramelized. To assist soften the fennel and keep it from sticking, you may add a little water if necessary.

In a bowl, mix together the eggs, turmeric powder, infused saffron (with water), and a sprinkle of salt, if needed, until well blended.

Cook the omelet by pushing the caramelized fennel to one side of the griddle. Spread the egg mixture equally on the other side of the pan after pouring it in. Cook until the edges start to set, approximately 3 to 4 minutes.

Cook the omelet for one more minute, or until the eggs are set, after gently folding it in half over the fennel. Place the omelet on a platter and add some fresh herbs as a garnish.

Warm up and serve.

Black Garlic and Shiitake Mushroom Bowl

(per serving)

Serving Size: 1 bowl

Calories: 290

Fats: 20g

Carbs: 10g

Protein: 18g

Sugars: 1g

Gluten-Free: Yes

Dairy-Free: Yes

Vegan: No (contains eggs)

2 large eggs

2 cloves black garlic, minced

1 cup shiitake mushrooms, sliced

1 tablespoon olive oil (or coconut oil)

Salt, to taste (optional and based on individual dietary needs)

Fresh microgreens, for garnish

Heat the olive oil in a pan over medium heat. After adding the sliced shiitake mushrooms, cook them for five to seven minutes, or until they are soft and beginning to become golden.

To avoid burning, add the minced black garlic to the pan and simmer for a further one to two minutes, stirring often.

Whisk the eggs in a bowl. Add the eggs, black garlic, and mushrooms to the skillet. Cook, stirring gently, for 3–4 minutes, or until the eggs are scrambled and just set.

Add a bit of salt if you'd like. Take off the heat and pour the mixture into a basin. Garnish with fresh microgreens on top.

Warm up and serve as a light dinner or a healthy breakfast.

Astragalus Root and Duck Egg Omelet

(per serving)

Serving Size: 1 omelet

Calories: 450

Fats: 30g

Carbs: 8g

Protein: 35g

Sugars: 1g (naturally occurring)

Gluten-Free: Yes

Dairy-Free: Yes

Vegan: No (due to eggs)

3 duck eggs

1 teaspoon astragalus powder

1/4 cup chives, finely chopped

1 cup wild mushrooms, sliced (e.g. chanterelles, morels, or any AIP-friendly variety)

1 tablespoon olive oil (or coconut oil)

Salt to taste (optional and in moderation for AIP)

In a pan over medium heat, heat the olive oil. After adding the sliced wild mushrooms, cook them for five to seven minutes, or until they are soft and have a light brown. Take off the heat and put it aside.

Break the duck eggs in a bowl and whisk in the chopped chives and astragalus powder until well blended.

To prepare the omelet, put the egg mixture in the same pan and heat it to medium-low. Cook until the edges start to set, approximately 2 to 3 minutes.

Gently add the sautéed wild mushrooms to one side of the omelet after the edges have set.

The remaining half of the omelet should be carefully folded over the mushrooms and cooked for a further two to three minutes, or until the eggs are cooked to your preferred consistency.

Transfer the heated omelet to a dish.

Golden Milk Scrambled Eggs

(per serving)

Serving Size: 2 scrambled eggs

Calories: 320

Fats: 25g

Carbs: 6g

Protein: 18g

Sugars: 2g

Gluten-Free: Yes

Dairy-Free: Yes

Vegan: No (contains eggs)

4 large eggs

1/4 cup coconut milk (full-fat for creaminess)

1 teaspoon ground turmeric

1/2 teaspoon fresh ginger, grated or 1/4 teaspoon ground ginger

1/4 teaspoon black pepper (optional, omit for strict AIP)

Salt to taste (optional, use a pinch of sea salt or omit for strict AIP)

1 tablespoon coconut oil (or other AIP-friendly oil for cooking)

Beat the eggs, coconut milk, ginger, turmeric, black pepper (if using), and salt in a bowl until well blended.

Melt the coconut oil in a non-stick skillet over medium heat.

Fill the skillet with the egg mixture. Allow it to settle for a few minutes, then use a spatula to gently stir, moving the eggs from the sides to the middle.

Keep cooking, stirring gently, for 3–4 minutes, or until the eggs are cooked through but still soft and creamy.

Take off the heat and serve right away. Savor the warm golden milk scrambled eggs.

Matcha Green Tea Egg White Bowl

(per serving)

Serving Size: 1 bowl

Calories: 100

Fats: 3g

Carbs: 2g

Protein: 18g

Sugars: 0g

Gluten-Free: Yes

Dairy-Free: Yes

Vegan: No (due to egg whites)

4 large egg whites

1 teaspoon matcha powder

1 tablespoon water

1 sheet nori, cut into small strips

1 teaspoon sesame seeds (optional, ensure they are compliant with your dietary needs)

Beat the egg whites in a mixing dish until they are foamy and have slightly grown in volume.

Whisk the matcha powder and water in a small bowl until smooth.

The matcha mixture should be gently folded into the whipped egg whites until it is completely incorporated. Take care not to deflate the egg whites too much.

Heat a non-stick skillet over medium-low heat after lightly coating it with oil (optional). Fill the skillet with the matcha mixture and egg white. Cook until the sides begin to firm, approximately 2 to 3 minutes. Carefully turn and cook for another 2 minutes, or until cooked through.

Pour the egg white matcha mixture onto a bowl after it's done. If using, sprinkle sesame seeds and nori strips over top.

Sardine and Olive Antiox Bowl

(per serving)

Serving Size: 1 bowl

Calories: 380

Fats: 27g

Carbs: 6g

Protein: 30g

Sugars: 1g (naturally occurring)

Gluten-Free: Yes

Dairy-Free: Yes

Vegan: No

2 large eggs

1 can sardines in olive oil (about 100g), drained

1/4 cup kalamata olives, pitted and chopped

1 tablespoon capers, rinsed and drained

1 tablespoon fresh parsley, chopped

1 tablespoon fresh dill or basil, chopped

Salt and pepper to taste (optional, use sparingly or omit for AIP)

Put the eggs in a small saucepan and add water to cover them. Place over medium heat and bring to a boil. For hard-boiled eggs, lower the heat to low and simmer for 9 to 12 minutes after it has boiled. Take off the heat, place in an ice bath, and allow it to cool for five minutes. Peel and put aside.

Put the chopped kalamata olives, capers, and drained sardines in a serving dish.

Top the sardine and olive mixture with the chopped parsley and dill (or basil).

Top the sardine and olive mixture with the cooked eggs, cut in half.

Season with salt and pepper to taste (optional), and drizzle with a little olive oil if you'd like.

Liver and Onion Healing Bowl

(per serving)

Serving Size: 1 bowl

Calories: 430

Fats: 28g

Carbohydrates: 18g

Protein: 36g

Sugars: 6g (naturally occurring)

Gluten-Free: Yes

Dairy-Free: Yes

Vegan: No (contains eggs and liver)

200g beef or chicken liver, cleaned and sliced

2 large eggs

1 large onion, thinly sliced

2 tablespoons olive oil or coconut oil

Fresh thyme leaves (to taste)

Salt (to taste, optional)

Pepper (to taste, optional)

Heat 1 tablespoon of coconut or olive oil in a big pan over medium heat.

Saute the sliced onions for ten to fifteen minutes, or until they are soft and caramelized, adding a touch of salt if needed. Stir from time to time to avoid scorching. After taking the onions out of the pan, put them aside.

Pour the last tablespoon of oil into the same skillet. Raise the temperature to medium-high.

Cook the liver slices in the pan for 3–4 minutes on each side, or until they are browned and cooked through. To preserve softness, don't overcook.

In the last minute of cooking, add salt, pepper (if using), and fresh thyme.

While the liver is cooking, prepare the eggs in a different pan to your preferred consistency (fried, poached, or scrambled).

Put the fried eggs on top of the caramelized onions and sautéed liver in a bowl.

If preferred, garnish with more fresh thyme..

Stinging Nettle Spring Omelet

(per serving)

Serving Size: 1 omelet

Calories: 350

Fats: 26g

Carbohydrates: 8g

Protein: 19g

Sugars: 1g

Gluten-Free: Yes

Dairy-Free: No (if goat cheese is included; omit for strict AIP)

Vegan: No

2 large eggs

1 cup blanched stinging nettles, chopped (fresh or frozen)

1/4 cup goat cheese, crumbled (optional for AIP)

2 tablespoons pine nuts

Salt and pepper to taste (omit if strictly following AIP)

1 tablespoon olive oil or coconut oil (for cooking)

Blanch the stinging nettles in boiling water for two to three minutes until they wilt if you are using fresh nettles. After draining, chill with cold water. Chop and reserve.

Beat the eggs in a bowl until they are well blended. If using, add salt and pepper.

In a non-stick skillet, heat the coconut oil or olive oil over medium heat. Add the whisked eggs and heat until the edges begin to firm, approximately 1 to 2 minutes.

Gently raise the omelet's edges so that any eggs that aren't cooked may run below. Add the chopped nettles, goat cheese, and pine nuts to

one side of the omelet when the bottom is set but the top is still somewhat runny.

Over the contents, carefully fold the omelet in half. Continue cooking for one more minute, or until the omelet is cooked through and the cheese has melted somewhat.

Serve the omelet warm after sliding it onto a dish.

Green Plantain and Cricket Flour Pancakes

(per serving, makes about 4 pancakes)

Serving Size: 2 pancakes

Calories: 310

Fats: 12g

Carbohydrates: 40g

Protein: 10g

Sugars: 2g (naturally occurring from plantains)

Gluten-Free: Yes

Dairy-Free: Yes

Vegan: No (due to eggs)

2 medium green plantains, peeled and chopped

1/2 cup cricket flour

2 large eggs

1 teaspoon vanilla extract

1/2 teaspoon ground cinnamon

1/4 teaspoon salt

1-2 tablespoons coconut oil (for cooking)

Cook the chopped green plantains in a saucepan of boiling water for about 15 minutes, or until they are soft. After draining, let it cool somewhat.

Put the cooked plantains, cricket flour, eggs, vanilla essence, cinnamon, and salt in a food processor or blender. Blend until the batter is smooth.

Heat 1 tablespoon of coconut oil in a non-stick pan over medium heat.

For each pancake, add 1/4 cup of batter to the skillet. Cook until bubbles appear on the surface, approximately 3–4 minutes. Cook for a further two to three minutes after flipping, or until golden brown.

Repeat with the remaining batter, using more coconut oil as necessary.

Top with your preferred AIP-friendly ingredients, such fresh fruit or coconut yogurt, and serve warm.

Tiger Nut and Water Chestnut Muffins

(per muffin, makes about 8 muffins)

Serving Size: 1 muffin

Calories: 150

Fats: 7g

Carbs: 21g

Protein: 3g

Sugars: 6g (naturally occurring from honey and water chestnuts)

Gluten-Free: Yes

Dairy-Free: Yes

Vegan: No (contains eggs)

1 cup tiger nut flour

1/2 cup water chestnuts, finely chopped

2 large eggs

1/4 cup honey (adjust based on sweetness preference)

1 teaspoon vanilla extract

1/2 teaspoon baking soda

1/4 teaspoon salt

1/4 cup coconut oil, melted (or any AIP-friendly oil)

First, preheat the oven to 350°F (175°C). Next, grease or line a muffin tray with paper liners.

Put the baking soda, salt, and tiger nut flour in a large basin.

In a separate dish, mix together the eggs, honey, vanilla extract, and melted coconut oil until well blended.

In the fourth step, the wet components are added to the dry ingredients and mixed until they are barely incorporated. Add the chopped water chestnuts and fold gently.

Fill each muffin cup approximately two-thirds of the way to the top with batter.

A toothpick inserted in the middle should come out clean after 18 to 20 minutes of baking in a preheated oven.

After a few minutes of cooling in the muffin tray, move the muffins to a wire rack to finish cooling. Have fun!

Cassava and Collagen Protein Pancakes

(per serving, makes about 4 pancakes)

Serving Size: 2 pancakes

Calories: 260

Fats: 14g

Carbs: 28g

Protein: 10g

Sugars: 2g (naturally occurring)

Gluten-Free: Yes

Dairy-Free: Yes

Vegan: No (contains eggs)

1 cup cassava flour

1/4 cup collagen peptides

2 large eggs

3/4 cup coconut milk (canned or carton)

1 teaspoon ground cinnamon

1/2 teaspoon baking powder (optional, for fluffiness)

Pinch of salt

Coconut oil or ghee (for cooking)

In a large bowl, mix together the baking powder (if using), powdered cinnamon, collagen peptides, cassava flour, and salt.

Whisk the eggs and coconut milk in another bowl. Stir this liquid into the dry ingredients until smooth and well blended.

Place a non-stick skillet over medium heat and lightly coat it with ghee or coconut oil.

For each pancake, add around 1/4 cup of batter to the skillet. Cook until bubbles appear on the surface, approximately 2 to 3 minutes. Cook for 1-2 more minutes after flipping, or until golden brown.

Then, take it out of the pan and serve it warm. Savor it on its own or with AIP-compliant garnishes like honey or fresh fruit.

Japanese Yam Purple Muffins

(per muffin, makes about 12 muffins)

Serving Size: 1 muffin

Calories: 130

Fats: 5g

Carbs: 18g

Protein: 3g

Sugars: 5g (naturally occurring from maple syrup and yam)

1 cup purple yam, cooked and mashed (about 200g)

1 cup coconut flour

4 large eggs

1/4 cup maple syrup

1 teaspoon vanilla extract

1/2 teaspoon baking soda

1/2 teaspoon salt

1/2 teaspoon ground cinnamon (optional)

Gluten-Free: Yes

Dairy-Free: Yes

Vegan: No (contains eggs)

The first step is to preheat the oven to 350°F (175°C). Grease a muffin tray gently or line it with paper liners.

Steam or boil the purple yam until it is soft. After letting it cool, mash it until it's smooth.

Put the mashed purple yam, eggs, coconut flour, maple syrup, baking soda, vanilla extract, salt, and ground cinnamon (if using) in a large mixing basin.

Stir until a thick batter forms and everything is fully incorporated. To give the coconut flour time to absorb the liquid, let the batter rest for about five minutes.

Using a spoon, fill each muffin tin cup approximately 3/4 of the way to the top.

Bake until a toothpick inserted in the middle comes out clean, 20 to 25 minutes.

Let the muffins cool in the muffin tray for a couple of minutes, then move them to a wire rack to finish cooling.

Chestnut and Carob Breakfast Muffins

(per muffin, recipe yields about 6 muffins)

Serving Size: 1 muffin

Calories: 160

Fats: 6g

Carbohydrates: 24g

Protein: 4g

Sugars: 7g (naturally occurring from banana and honey)

Gluten-Free: Yes

Dairy-Free: Yes

Vegan: No (contains eggs, but you can substitute with flax eggs if needed)

1 cup chestnut flour

1/4 cup carob powder

2 large eggs

1 ripe banana, mashed

2 tablespoons honey (optional, adjust to taste)

1/2 teaspoon baking soda

1/4 teaspoon salt

1/4 teaspoon cinnamon (optional, for added flavor)

Preheat the oven to 350°F (175°C). Lightly oil or line a muffin pan with paper liners.

Put the baking soda, cinnamon (if using), carob powder, chestnut flour, and salt in a big basin. Mix well by whisking.

Beat the eggs, honey, and mashed banana in a separate bowl until smooth.

In the fourth step, the wet components are added to the dry ingredients and stirred until they are barely blended. A few lumps are OK; do not overmix.

Fill each muffin cup approximately 3/4 of the way to the top with batter.

A toothpick put into the middle of a muffin should come out clean after 20 to 25 minutes of baking in a preheated oven.

After 5 minutes of cooling in the pan, move the muffins to a wire rack to finish cooling.

Green Banana Resistant Starch Pancakes

(per serving, 2 pancakes)

Serving Size: 2 pancakes

Calories: 250

Fats: 9g

Carbs: 36g

Protein: 6g

Sugars: 3g (naturally occurring from ingredients)

Gluten-Free: Yes

Dairy-Free: Yes

Vegan: No (due to eggs)

1 cup green banana flour

2 large eggs

1 cup coconut milk (full-fat or light, unsweetened)

1 teaspoon vanilla extract

1 teaspoon cinnamon (optional)

Pinch of salt

Coconut oil or ghee for cooking

In a large bowl, mix together the eggs, coconut milk, green banana flour, cinnamon, vanilla essence, and salt until smooth and well blended.

Preheat a non-stick skillet or griddle to medium heat. Grease the pan with a little coconut oil or ghee.

For each pancake, pour about 1/4 cup of batter into the griddle. Cook for two to three minutes, or until the edges seem firm and bubbles appear on the top. Cook for a further two to three minutes after flipping, or until golden brown.

While you cook the rest of the batter, take the pancakes out of the skillet and keep them warm. Serve with your preferred AIP-friendly garnishes, including fresh fruit or, if you'd like, a honey drizzle.

Lotus Root and Almond Flour Muffins

(per muffin, makes about 12 muffins)

Serving Size: 1 muffin

Calories: 150

Fats: 10g

Carbs: 15g

Protein: 4g

Sugars: 6g (naturally occurring from honey and lotus root)

Gluten-Free: Yes

Dairy-Free: Yes

Vegan: No (due to eggs)

1 cup ground lotus root (fresh or frozen, cooked and pureed)

2 cups almond flour

3 large eggs

1/4 cup honey (or to taste)

1 teaspoon fresh ginger, grated

1/2 teaspoon baking soda

1/4 teaspoon salt

Preheat the oven to 350°F (175°C). Lightly oil or line a muffin pan with paper liners.

If you're using fresh lotus root, peel and cut it into slices, then steam or boil it for 15 to 20 minutes to make it soft. Puree the lotus root until it's smooth after it has cooled.

Put the almond flour, eggs, honey, grated ginger, baking soda, salt, and powdered lotus root puree in a big basin. Blend until smooth and fully mixed.

Fill each muffin tin cup approximately two-thirds of the way to the top with batter.

The muffins should be golden brown and a toothpick inserted in the middle should come out clean after 20 to 25 minutes of baking in a preheated oven.

After allowing the muffins to cool in the pan for about five minutes, move them to a wire rack to finish cooling..

Breadfruit Flour Morning Pancakes

(per serving, recipe yields about 4 pancakes)

Serving Size: 2 pancakes

Calories: 300

Fats: 18g

Carbs: 32g

Protein: 6g

Sugars: 2g (naturally occurring from coconut milk)

Gluten-Free: Yes

Dairy-Free: Yes

Vegan: No (due to eggs)

1 cup breadfruit flour

2 large eggs

1 cup coconut milk (canned or fresh)

1 teaspoon vanilla extract

1/2 teaspoon ground nutmeg

1 tablespoon coconut oil (for cooking)

Put the breadfruit flour and powdered nutmeg in a big basin.

Beat the eggs, coconut milk, and vanilla extract in a separate dish until well blended.

Mix the dry ingredients until they are smooth by pouring the liquid components into them. You may adjust the batter's consistency by adding a little more coconut milk if it's too thick.

Over medium heat, add coconut oil to a non-stick skillet or griddle and let it melt, coating the pan.

For each pancake, pour about 1/4 cup of batter into the skillet. Cook until bubbles appear on the top, approximately 2 to 3 minutes. Then, turn and cook for another 2 to 3 minutes, or until golden brown.

Present warm, garnished with your preferred toppings, including fresh fruit, coconut yogurt, or honey (if preferred)..

Taro Root Purple Muffins

(per muffin, makes about 12 muffins)

Serving Size: 1 muffin

Calories: 140

Fats: 6g

Carbs: 19g

Protein: 4g

Sugars: 4g (naturally occurring from maple syrup)

Gluten-Free: Yes

Dairy-Free: Yes

Vegan: No (contains eggs)

1 cup taro flour

1/2 cup coconut flour

3 large eggs

1/4 cup maple syrup

1 teaspoon vanilla extract

1/2 teaspoon baking soda

1/2 teaspoon salt

1/2 cup water (adjust as needed for batter consistency)

First, preheat the oven to 350°F (175°C). Next, lubricate a muffin tray with coconut oil or fill it with paper liners.

Put the taro flour, coconut flour, baking soda, and salt in a big basin.

Whisk the eggs, water, maple syrup, and vanilla essence in a separate basin.

Stir the dry ingredients until well incorporated, then gradually add the liquid mixture. A tablespoon of water at a time may be added to the batter if it's too thick until the right consistency is achieved.

Fill each muffin tin cup approximately 3/4 of the way to the top with batter.

A toothpick put into the middle of a muffin should come out clean after 20 to 25 minutes of baking in a preheated oven.

After 5 minutes of cooling in the muffin tray, move the muffins to a wire rack to finish cooling.

Mesquite and Tigernut Pancakes

(per serving, makes about 4 pancakes)

Serving Size: 2 pancakes

Calories: 320

Fats: 12g

Carbs: 45g

Protein: 10g

Sugars: 5g (naturally occurring from honey and other ingredients)

Gluten-Free: Yes

Dairy-Free: Yes

Vegan: No (contains eggs; can substitute with a flax egg for a vegan option)

1/2 cup mesquite flour

1/2 cup tigernut flour

2 large eggs

1 cup unsweetened almond milk

1 teaspoon ground cinnamon

1 tablespoon honey (optional, adjust to taste)

Pinch of salt

Coconut oil (for cooking)

Put the tigernut flour, mesquite flour, ground cinnamon, and salt in a mixing basin. Whisk the eggs, almond milk, and honey (if using) in another bowl. Stirring until well blended, gradually add the wet components to the dry ingredients. The batter needs to be pourable and smooth.

Preheat a non-stick skillet or griddle to medium heat. Lightly grease the pan's surface with coconut oil.

For each pancake, add around 1/4 cup of batter to the skillet. Cook for two to three minutes, or until bubbles appear on the top, then turn and continue cooking for one to two minutes more, or until cooked through and golden brown.

To serve, take it out of the pan and keep it warm while you continue with the rest of the batter. Top the pancakes with your preferred toppings (such maple syrup or fresh fruit) and serve them warm.

Soups and Stews for Healing

Turmeric-Ginger Chicken Bone Broth

(per serving, assuming 6 servings)

Serving Size: 1 cup

Calories: 60

Fats: 2g

Carbs: 3g

Protein: 9g

Sugars: 0g

Gluten-Free: Yes

Dairy-Free: Yes

Vegan: No (as it contains chicken bones)

2 pounds chicken bones (preferably organic)

1 tablespoon turmeric powder

1 tablespoon fresh ginger, sliced

2 stalks lemongrass, chopped

2-3 kaffir lime leaves

1 onion, quartered

2-3 cloves garlic, crushed

10 cups water

Salt to taste (optional and use sparingly for AIP)

Put the chicken bones, water, chopped lemongrass, kaffir lime leaves, turmeric powder, fresh ginger, onion, and garlic in a big saucepan.

Heat the mixture on high until it boils.

Cover, lower the heat to low, and simmer for 6-8 hours. You may simmer for up to 24 hours for a deeper taste.

After the broth has simmered, turn off the heat and allow it to cool a little. Pour the broth into a large dish using a fine-mesh strainer, discarding the solids.

If you like, add salt after tasting the soup.

Allow the broth to cool fully before storing it in the fridge for up to five days in sealed containers or freezing it for extended storage. It may also be served warm as a filling beverage.

Wild-Caught Fish Head Soup

(per serving, assuming 4 servings)

Serving Size: 1 bowl of soup

Calories: 150

Fats: 8g

Carbs: 5g

Protein: 18g

Sugars: 1g

Gluten-Free: Yes

Dairy-Free: Yes

Vegan: No (due to fish heads)

AIP-Friendly: Yes

2 wild-caught fish heads (salmon or snapper)

6 cups water

1 cup seaweed (dried wakame for kombu)

1 tablespoon fresh ginger, sliced

3 green onions, chopped (white and green parts separated)

1 tablespoon olive oil or coconut oil

Salt to taste (omit if strictly AIP)

1 tablespoon apple cider vinegar (optional)

The first step is to prepare the seaweed. If you are using dried seaweed, soak it in water for ten to fifteen minutes until it softens. After draining, put away.

Heat the coconut or olive oil in a big saucepan over medium heat.

Add the white portions of the green onions and the sliced ginger to the saucepan. Sauté until aromatic, approximately 2 to 3 minutes.

Put the water into the pot with the fish heads. Reduce to a simmer after bringing to a boil.

Skim any froth that comes to the top of the soup and let it simmer for 30 to 40 minutes.

After simmering, add the green portions of the green onions and the soaked seaweed. Add apple cider vinegar if using. Simmer for a further five to ten minutes.

Adjust the seasoning according to taste. Take off the heat and serve warm.

Oxtail and Herb Bone Broth

(per serving, based on 8 servings)

Serving Size: 1 cup broth

Calories: 150

Fats: 10g

Carbs: 1g

Protein: 12g

Sugars: 0g

Gluten-Free: Yes

Dairy-Free: Yes

Vegan: No (contains meat)

2 pounds oxtail

2 tablespoons apple cider vinegar

8 cups filtered water

2-3 fresh bay leaves

2-3 sprigs fresh thyme

1 medium onion, quartered

2-3 cloves garlic, smashed

1 teaspoon salt (adjust to taste)

Optional: 1-2 carrots, chopped (for added flavor)

To prepare the oxtail, rinse it in cold water. Use paper towels to pat dry.

Add the oxtail, apple cider vinegar, filtered water, bay leaves, thyme, onion, garlic, salt, and optional carrots to a large stockpot.

The mixture should be brought to a boil over medium-high heat

Lower the heat to low, partly cover, and simmer for eight to twelve hours. The taste will become richer the longer it simmers.

Take the oxtail and herbs out of the saucepan after it's cooked. To get rid of the particles, strain the broth using cheesecloth or a fine-mesh sieve.

Before putting the broth in the fridge or freezer, let it cool. As it cools, the fat will rise to the top and may be skimmed off if preferred.

Lamb Neck Broth with Moroccan Spices

(per serving, based on 8 servings)

Serving Size: 1 cup

Calories: 150

Fats: 10g

Carbs: 5g

Protein: 13g

Sugars: 1g

Gluten-Free: Yes

Dairy-Free: Yes

AIP-Compliant: Yes

2 lbs lamb neck bones

1 onion, chopped

2 carrots, chopped

2 celery stalks, chopped

4 cloves garlic, smashed

1-inch piece of fresh ginger, sliced

1 tablespoon olive oil

8 cups water

1 teaspoon ground cumin

1 teaspoon ground coriander

1 teaspoon ground turmeric

1/2 teaspoon ground cinnamon

1/2 teaspoon ground black pepper (omit for strict AIP)

Salt to taste

Fresh cilantro or parsley for garnish (optional)

To sauté vegetables, heat olive oil in a large saucepan over medium heat. Add the chopped celery, carrots, and onion and sauté for 5 to 7 minutes, or until they start to soften.

Cook for another 2 minutes until aromatic, stirring in the sliced ginger and crushed garlic.

Add the ground cumin, coriander, turmeric, cinnamon, and black pepper (if using) to the saucepan after adding the lamb neck bones. Coat the bones with the seasonings by stirring.

Bring the mixture to a boil by adding 8 cups of water. For three to four hours, simmer uncovered over low heat.

To maintain the broth's clarity, periodically skim any foam that accumulates on the top.

Turn off the heat after the broth has simmered. Remove the sediments from the broth by straining it through a fine-mesh screen into a large dish or another saucepan.

Add salt to the broth. If preferred, top with fresh parsley or cilantro and serve hot.

Roasted Kabocha Squash Soup

(per serving)

Serving Size: 1 cup (approx. 1/6 of the soup)

Calories: 250

Fats: 18g

Carbs: 22g

Protein: 3g

Sugars: 4g (naturally occurring)

Gluten-Free: Yes

Dairy-Free: Yes

Vegan: Yes

1 medium kabocha squash (about 2-3 pounds), halved and seeds removed

2 tablespoons olive oil (or avocado oil)

1 medium onion, diced

3 cloves garlic, minced

4 cups vegetable broth (ensure it's AIP-compliant)

1 teaspoon fresh sage, chopped or ½ teaspoon dried sage

1 can (13.5 oz) coconut cream

Salt and pepper to taste (omit if strictly AIP)

Optional garnishes: Additional coconut cream, fresh sage leaves

First, roast the squash: Set the oven temperature to 400°F, or 200°C. Place the halves of kabocha squash cut-side down on a baking pan after drizzling them with 1 tablespoon of olive oil. Roast until the meat is tender, approximately 40 to 50 minutes. Scoop the meat into a dish after letting it cool a little.

Heat the remaining tablespoon of olive oil in a big saucepan over medium heat. Add the chopped onion and cook for 5 to 7 minutes, or until it becomes transparent. Cook for a further one to two minutes, or until aromatic, after adding the minced garlic and fresh sage.

Pour the veggie stock into the saucepan and add the roasted kabocha squash. To allow the flavors to mingle, bring to a simmer and stew for ten to fifteen minutes.

Blend the soup with an immersion blender until it's smooth. As an alternative, pour the soup into a blender in small portions and process until it becomes smooth.

If required, adjust the seasoning with salt and pepper after stirring in the coconut cream. Give it a few minutes to heat through.

If preferred, top the soup with more coconut cream and fresh sage leaves after ladling it into bowls..

Watercress and Daikon Radish Detox Soup

(per serving)

Serving Size: 1 cup

Calories: 60

Fats: 2g

Carbs: 12g

Protein: 2g

Sugars: 2g

Gluten-Free: Yes

Dairy-Free: Yes

Vegan: Yes

1 tablespoon olive oil (optional)

1 medium daikon radish, peeled and diced

1 small onion, diced (use a green onion for AIP)

2 cloves garlic, minced

4 cups vegetable broth (low-sodium, AIP-compliant)

2 cups watercress, rinsed and chopped

1 medium carrot, diced

1 teaspoon fresh ginger, grated

Salt and pepper to taste (use AIP-friendly seasonings)

Juice of 1 lime (for serving)

Heat the olive oil in a large saucepan over medium heat. Add the chopped garlic, onion (or green onion), and daikon radish. The onion should be transparent after approximately five minutes of sautéing.

Add water and veggie broth. Add the grated ginger and chopped carrot. Reduce heat to a simmer after bringing to a boil.

Simmer the soup until the carrots and daikon are soft, approximately 20 minutes.

Add the chopped watercress and cook until it wilts, about 5 more minutes.

You may purée the soup to the consistency you want with an immersion blender for a smoother texture.

Before serving, pour in some lime juice and season with salt and pepper to taste..

Pureed Celeriac and Fennel Soup

(per serving)

Serving Size: 1 cup

Calories: 150

Fats: 10g

Carbs: 15g

Protein: 3g

Sugars: 2g

Gluten-Free: Yes

Dairy-Free: Yes

Vegan: Yes

1 medium celeriac (celery root), peeled and diced

1 large fennel bulb, sliced (reserve some fronds for garnish)

1 medium onion, chopped

2 cloves garlic, minced

4 cups vegetable broth (low-sodium)

2 tablespoons olive oil

1 tablespoon truffle oil (adjust to taste)

Salt and pepper to taste (use salt alternatives if needed)

Fresh herbs for garnish (optional)

The first step is to sauté aromatics by heating olive oil in a big saucepan over medium heat. Sauté the minced garlic and chopped onion for around five minutes, or until they are aromatic and tender.

Add the sliced fennel and chopped celeriac to the saucepan and stir to mix. Allow the veggies to soften by cooking for a further five minutes.

Add the veggie broth and heat until it boils. Lower the heat and simmer for 20 to 25 minutes, or until the veggies are soft.

Carefully purée the soup with an immersion blender or a standard blender until it is creamy and smooth.

Season with salt and pepper to taste and stir in the truffle oil. If preferred, top with more truffle oil and garnish with the saved fennel fronds before serving hot..

Japanese-Style Taro Root and Seaweed Soup

(per serving)

Serving Size: 1 bowl (approximately 1.5 cups)

Calories: 150

Fats: 1g

Carbohydrates: 36g

Protein: 3g

Sugars: 1g

Gluten-Free: Yes

Dairy-Free: Yes

Vegan: Yes

2 cups taro root, peeled and diced

4 cups water or vegetable broth (ensure it's AIP-compliant)

1/2 cup dried seaweed (wakame or similar), soaked and chopped

1 tablespoon fresh ginger, grated

2 green onions, chopped (green parts only)

1 tablespoon coconut aminos

Salt to taste (optional)

To prepare the seaweed, soak it in water for ten to fifteen minutes until it becomes pliable. Chop and drain.

Put the chopped taro root and water or vegetable broth in a big saucepan. Reduce to a simmer after bringing to a boil over medium heat. Cook until the taro is soft, approximately 15 to 20 minutes.

Add the grated ginger, coconut aminos, and the soaked and sliced seaweed once the taro is soft. Simmer for five to seven more minutes.

If desired, add salt to taste and adjust seasoning.

The soup may be served hot by ladling it into bowls and topping them with chopped green onions..

Roasted Parsnip and Wild Mushroom

(per serving)

Serving Size: 1 cup

Calories: 150

Fats: 5g

Carbs: 25g

Protein: 3g

Sugars: 4g (naturally occurring from vegetables)

Gluten-Free: Yes

Dairy-Free: Yes

Vegan: Yes

2 cups parsnips, peeled and diced

2 cups wild mushrooms (such as shiitake, oyster, or cremini), chopped

1 medium onion, chopped

3 cloves garlic, minced

4 cups vegetable broth (low-sodium, AIP-compliant)

2 tablespoons olive oil

1 tablespoon fresh thyme, chopped

1 tablespoon fresh parsley, chopped

Salt and pepper, to taste (omit salt for strict AIP)

Optional: A squeeze of lemon juice for brightness

Set the oven temperature to 400°F (200°C).

Combine the chopped mushrooms and diced parsnips with olive oil, salt, and pepper on a baking sheet. They should be soft and faintly browned after 25 to 30 minutes of roasting in a single layer.

Heat a little amount of olive oil in a big saucepan over medium heat. Add the chopped onion and cook for about five minutes, or until it becomes transparent. Sauté for one more minute after adding the minced garlic.

Add the roasted parsnips and mushrooms to the saucepan with the garlic and onions. Add the fresh thyme and the veggie broth. Cook for ten to fifteen minutes after bringing to a simmer.

Blend the soup with an immersion blender until it's creamy and smooth. (Alternatively, carefully handle the boiling liquid while transferring the soup in batches to a blender.)

Add the fresh parsley and, if you'd like, adjust the flavor with lemon juice, salt, and pepper.

Ladle the soup into bowls and, if you'd like, top with more herbs..

Grass-Fed Beef Tongue Stew

(per serving, makes approximately 4 servings)

Serving Size: 1 bowl of stew

Calories: 360

Fats: 18g

Carbs: 30g

Protein: 25g

Sugars: 6g

Gluten-Free: Yes

Dairy-Free: Yes

AIP-Friendly: Yes (omit black pepper and any non-AIP herbs)

1 lb grass-fed beef tongue, cleaned and trimmed

2 tablespoons olive oil (or coconut oil)

1 medium onion, diced

3 cloves garlic, minced

2 medium carrots, peeled and diced

2 medium parsnips, peeled and diced

2 medium sweet potatoes, peeled and cubed

4 cups beef broth (low-sodium)

1 teaspoon dried thyme

1 teaspoon dried oregano

1 bay leaf

Salt and pepper to taste (omit pepper for strict AIP)

Fresh parsley, chopped (for garnish)

Bring the beef tongue to a boil in a big saucepan with water covering it. Simmer until tender, approximately 2 hours. Peel off the skin after removing the tongue and letting it cool. Slice the tongue into small pieces.

Heat the olive oil in the same saucepan over medium heat. Sauté the chopped onion and garlic for around five minutes, or until they become transparent.

Put the sweet potatoes, carrots, and parsnips in the saucepan. Cook, stirring occasionally, for a further 5 to 7 minutes.

Put back into the pot the cooked beef tongue. Add the bay leaf, oregano, thyme, and beef broth, and season with salt (and pepper, if using).

Reduce the heat to low after bringing the stew to a boil. For about forty-five minutes, or until the flavors are thoroughly blended and the veggies are soft, cover and simmer.

Before serving, take out the bay leaf. Add some freshly cut parsley as a garnish and dig in..

Wild Boar and Sweet Potato Stew

(per serving, serves 6)

Serving Size: 1 cup

Calories: 320

Fats: 10g

Carbs: 40g

Protein: 25g

Sugars: 7g (naturally occurring from vegetables)

Gluten-Free: Yes

Dairy-Free: Yes

Vegan: No

1.5 pounds wild boar, cubed (or substitute with lean pork if unavailable)

2 medium sweet potatoes, peeled and diced

1 medium onion, chopped

2 cloves garlic, minced

2 cups vegetable broth (AIP-compliant)

1 cup carrots, sliced

1 tablespoon fresh thyme, chopped

1 tablespoon fresh rosemary, chopped

1 tablespoon olive oil

Salt and pepper to taste (omit or reduce salt for strict AIP)

1 bay leaf

Heat the olive oil in a big saucepan or Dutch oven over medium-high heat. Sear the cubes of wild boar until they are browned on both sides. Set aside the meat after removing it.

Add the chopped garlic and onion to the same saucepan. The onion should be transparent after 3–4 minutes of sautéing.

Stir well after adding the chopped carrots and sweet potatoes to the saucepan.

Add the seared wild boar back to the saucepan after combining the ingredients. Season with salt and pepper to taste and add the vegetable broth, bay leaf, fresh thyme, and rosemary.

Reduce the heat to low after bringing the stew to a boil. Simmer, covered, until the wild boar is soft, approximately 1½ to 2 hours.

As needed, taste and modify the seasoning. Before serving, take out the bay leaf.

Ladle the stew into dishes and, if you'd like, top with some fresh herbs.

Rabbit and Turnip Stew with Fresh Bay Leaves

(per serving)

Serving Size: 1 bowl (approx. 1.5 cups)

Calories: 320

Fats: 12g

Carbs: 25g

Protein: 28g

Sugars: 5g

Gluten-Free: Yes

Dairy-Free: Yes

AIP-Friendly: Yes

2 pounds rabbit, cut into pieces

3 cups turnips, peeled and diced

1 large onion, chopped

3 cloves garlic, minced

4 cups vegetable broth (low-sodium)

2 tablespoons olive oil

1 tablespoon fresh thyme leaves

3-4 fresh bay leaves

Salt (to taste)

Pepper (to taste)

Heat the olive oil in a large saucepan or Dutch oven over medium-high heat. Add the rabbit pieces and cook for 5 to 7 minutes, or until browned on both sides. After removing the rabbit, put it aside.

Add the chopped garlic and onion to the same saucepan. Sauté for 3–4 minutes, or until the onion is transparent.

Put the rabbit back in the saucepan. Add the bay leaves, fresh thyme, vegetable broth, and chopped turnips. Mix to blend.

Reduce the heat to low after bringing the stew to a boil. The rabbit should be soft and cooked through after 1 to 2 hours of simmering under cover.

Taste the stew and adjust the seasoning with salt and pepper if necessary before serving. Before serving, take off the bay leaves.

The stew may be served warm by ladling it into bowls..

Sea Bass and Plantain Coconut Curry

(per serving, serves 4)

Serving Size: 1/4 of the recipe

Calories: 360

Fats: 20g

Carbs: 26g

Protein: 20g

Sugars: 5g

Gluten-Free: Yes

Dairy-Free: Yes

Vegan: No (due to fish)

1 pound sea bass filets (or any white fish)

1 medium ripe plantain, peeled and sliced

1 can (14 oz) coconut milk (full-fat)

1 tablespoon coconut oil

1 medium onion, chopped

2 cloves garlic, minced

1-inch piece of ginger, grated

1 tablespoon fresh lime juice

1 tablespoon curry powder (ensure AIP compliant)

Salt, to taste (use a pinch or omit if necessary)

Fresh cilantro, for garnish (optional)

Chop the onion, mince the ginger and garlic, and slice the plantain.

Heat coconut oil in a big skillet over medium heat. Sauté the chopped onion, ginger, and garlic for three to four minutes, or until the onion is transparent.

Incorporate the curry powder and the cut plantains. Allow the spices to roast by cooking for a further two minutes.

Add the coconut milk and mix well. Heat to a low simmer.

Submerge the sea bass filets in the coconut milk mixture in the pan. The fish should be cooked through and flake readily with a fork after 8 to 10 minutes of simmering.

Add the lime juice and salt to taste.

Take off the heat and, if you'd like, top with fresh cilantro. Warm up and serve..

Venison and Rutabaga Stew with Wild Mushrooms

(per serving)

Serving Size: 1 cup

Calories: 350

Fats: 15g

Carbs: 28g

Protein: 30g

Sugars: 4g

Gluten-Free: Yes

Dairy-Free: Yes

Vegan: No (contains venison)

1 lb venison stew meat, cut into 1-inch pieces

2 medium rutabagas, peeled and diced

1 cup wild mushrooms (e.g. chanterelles, morels), cleaned and sliced

1 large onion, diced

2 cloves garlic, minced

4 cups bone broth (beef or venison, homemade or store-bought)

2 carrots, diced

2 tablespoons olive oil or avocado oil

1 teaspoon dried thyme

1 teaspoon dried rosemary

Salt and pepper to taste (omit salt if strictly following AIP)

Fresh parsley, chopped (for garnish)

Heat the olive oil in a big saucepan or Dutch oven over medium heat. After 5 to 7 minutes, add the venison stew meat and brown it on both sides. Take out and put aside.

Add the chopped carrots and onion to the same saucepan. The onions should be transparent after around five minutes of sautéing. Cook the garlic for a further minute until it becomes aromatic.

Add the rutabaga and wild mushrooms and simmer for another 3 to 4 minutes, or until the mushrooms start to soften.

Put the venison back in the saucepan when it has browned. Stir in the dried rosemary, dry thyme, and bone broth. Heat the mixture until it boils.

Lower the heat to low, cover, and simmer until the rutabaga is cooked through and the venison is soft, approximately 1 to 2 hours.

Add salt and pepper (if using) to taste. Garnish with fresh parsley and serve hot..

Lunches and Light Meals

Roasted Fennel & Watercress Salad

(per serving)

Serving Size: 1 salad (approximately 1.5 cups)

Calories: 180

Fats: 10g

Carbs: 25g

Protein: 2g

Sugars: 12g (naturally occurring from figs)

Gluten-Free: Yes

Dairy-Free: Yes

Vegan: Yes

For the Salad:

2 medium fennel bulbs, sliced

1 tablespoon olive oil

Salt and pepper to taste (optional, can be omitted for strict AIP)

4 cups fresh watercress, washed and trimmed

For the Fig-Balsamic Dressing:

1/2 cup fresh figs, chopped

1/4 cup balsamic vinegar

1 tablespoon olive oil

1 teaspoon honey (optional, adjust to taste)

Salt to taste (optional, can be omitted for strict AIP)

The first step is to preheat the oven to 400°F (200°C).

Second, arrange the sliced fennel on a baking sheet and roast it.

Season with salt and pepper (if using) and drizzle with olive oil.

Stir the fennel halfway through and roast it in a warm oven for 25 to 30 minutes, or until it is soft and caramelized.

Add the olive oil, balsamic vinegar, and chopped figs to a small saucepan set over medium heat.

Cook, stirring constantly, until the figs are tender, approximately 5 to 7 minutes.

Take off the heat and combine with a conventional blender or an immersion blender until smooth. Add salt to taste and honey for sweetness if you'd like.

Put the fresh watercress and roasted fennel in a big dish.

Pour the fig-balsamic dressing over it and gently toss to mix.

Drizzle any leftover dressing over the salad after dividing it among plates. Serve right away.

Grilled Peach & Arugula Salad

(per serving, serves 4)

Serving Size: 1 salad

Calories: 180

Fats: 12g

Carbs: 20g

Protein: 2g

Sugars: 10g

Gluten-Free: Yes

Dairy-Free: Yes

Vegan: Yes (if using pure honey, otherwise omit for strict AIP)

For the Salad:

2 ripe peaches, halved and pitted

4 cups baby arugula

1/4 cup walnuts, toasted (optional, omit for strict AIP)

For the Lavender Honey Vinaigrette:

2 tablespoons olive oil

1 tablespoon lavender-infused honey (substitute with pure honey if strict AIP)

1 tablespoon apple cider vinegar

1 teaspoon dried lavender (culinary grade, optional)

Salt and pepper to taste (omit salt for strict AIP)

Turn the heat up to medium on your grill or grill pan.

To grill the peaches, lightly coat each half with olive oil. Put them on the grill cut-side down. The peaches should be soft and have grill marks after 3–4 minutes on the grill. Take off the heat and let it cool a little.

The vinaigrette is made by whisking together the olive oil, apple cider vinegar, lavender-infused honey, dried lavender (if using), salt, and pepper in a small basin.

Put the baby arugula and toasted walnuts (if using) in a big bowl. Add the grilled peaches to the salad after slicing them.

Drizzle the salad with the lavender honey vinaigrette and gently toss to mix.

Arrange the salad on plates and dig in!

Sea Vegetable & Cucumber Salad

(per serving)

Serving Size: Approximately 1 cup

Calories: 80

Fats: 4g

Carbs: 10g

Protein: 3g

Sugars: 2g (naturally occurring)

Gluten-Free: Yes

Dairy-Free: Yes

Vegan: Yes

For the Salad:

2 cups mixed seaweeds (wakame, dulse, or any AIP-friendly sea vegetables, rehydrated if dried)

1 large cucumber, thinly sliced

1/4 cup scallions, chopped (optional, use green tops only for AIP)

1/4 cup carrots, shredded (optional)

For the Ginger-Lime Dressing:

1 tablespoon fresh ginger, grated

Juice of 1 lime

1 tablespoon coconut aminos

1 tablespoon sesame oil (optional, use AIP-compliant oil if needed)

Salt to taste

If you're using dried seaweed, soak it in water for ten to fifteen minutes to rehydrate and soften it. If needed, drain and cut into bite-sized pieces.

To make the dressing, mix the grated ginger, lime juice, coconut aminos, sesame oil (if using), and salt in a small bowl and whisk until well blended.

In a big bowl, mix together the sliced cucumber, shredded carrots, onions, and rehydrated seaweeds.

Drizzle the salad with the ginger-lime dressing and gently toss to evenly coat all the ingredients.

Serve the salad right away after letting it rest for 5 to 10 minutes to allow the flavors to combine..

Roasted Beet & Microgreens Salad

(per serving)

Serving Size: 1 salad

Calories: 220

Fats: 10g

Carbs: 32g

Protein: 3g

Sugars: 12g (naturally occurring from beets and maple syrup)

Gluten-Free: Yes

Dairy-Free: Yes

Vegan: Yes

For the Salad:

2 medium rainbow beets, scrubbed and trimmed

2 cups fresh microgreens (such as arugula, sunflower, or radish)

1 tablespoon olive oil

Salt and pepper, to taste (omit if strictly AIP)

For the Maple-Cinnamon Dressing:

2 tablespoons pure maple syrup

1 tablespoon apple cider vinegar

1/2 teaspoon ground cinnamon

1 tablespoon olive oil

Salt, to taste (omit if strictly AIP)

The first step is to preheat the oven to 400°F (200°C).

Line a baking sheet with aluminum foil and wrap each beet separately.

Bake for 45 to 60 minutes, or until it is fork-tender. Take it out of the oven and let it cool a little.

Peel and cut the beets into wedges after they are cold enough to handle.

Whisk the olive oil, apple cider vinegar, maple syrup, and ground cinnamon in a small basin. If desired, add salt for seasoning.

To assemble the salad, place the roasted beet wedges on top of the fresh microgreens in a big bowl or serving tray.

Just before serving, drizzle the salad with the warm maple-cinnamon dressing.

Gently toss to mix, then serve right away.

Caramelized Pear & Endive Salad

(per serving, serves 4)

Serving Size: 1 salad serving

Calories: 200

Fats: 15g

Carbs: 24g

Protein: 2g

Sugars: 10g (naturally occurring from pears)

Gluten-Free: Yes

Dairy-Free: Yes

Vegan: Yes

Nut-Free: Omit walnuts if nut-free is required.

2 medium ripe pears, halved and cored

2 tablespoons olive oil (for roasting)

2 tablespoons rosemary-infused olive oil (see below for preparation)

2 heads Belgian endive, leaves separated

1/4 cup walnuts, chopped (optional for added crunch, if tolerated)

Salt and pepper to taste (use salt substitute if following strict AIP)

Rosemary-Infused Olive Oil

1/2 cup extra virgin olive oil

2-3 sprigs fresh rosemary

Get the Olive Oil Infused with Rosemary Ready:

Add the rosemary sprigs and 1/2 cup of olive oil to a small saucepan.

Allow the oil to infuse without boiling by heating over low heat for ten to fifteen minutes. Take off the heat and let it cool. Remove the rosemary using a strainer and save the oil.

Heat the oven to 400°F (200°C) in order to roast the pears.

Arrange the halved pears, cut side up, on a baking sheet. Season with salt (if using) and drizzle with 2 tablespoons olive oil.

Roast until soft and begin to caramelize, 20 to 25 minutes. Take it out of the oven and let it cool a little.

Put the salad together: Place the roasted pears (cut into wedges) and Belgian endive leaves in a large serving basin.

Pour over the olive oil flavored with rosemary.

Add walnuts, if using, and toss lightly to mix. To taste, add salt and pepper.

Serve right away as a side salad or light meal.

Wild-Caught Salmon & Fresh Herb Salad

(per serving)

Serving Size: 1 salad

Calories: 320

Fats: 21g

Carbs: 14g

Protein: 25g

Sugars: 3g (naturally occurring from vegetables and fruit)

Gluten-Free: Yes

Dairy-Free: Yes

Vegan: No

AIP Compliant: Yes (if not using black pepper)

For the Salad:

2 cups mixed greens (arugula, spinach, and kale)

1 cup flaked wild-caught salmon (cooked and cooled)

1/4 cup fresh parsley, chopped

1/4 cup fresh cilantro, chopped

1/4 cup fresh mint, chopped

1/4 cup cucumber, diced

1/4 cup radishes, thinly sliced (optional)

For the Citrus-Mint Dressing:

1/4 cup olive oil

Juice of 1 lemon

Juice of 1 orange

1 tablespoon fresh mint, finely chopped

Salt and pepper to taste (omit if strictly AIP)

Combine the olive oil, lemon juice, orange juice, and chopped mint in a small bowl and whisk to combine. To taste, add salt and pepper. Put aside.

Combine the flakes salmon, mixed greens, cucumber, radishes (if using), parsley, cilantro, mint, and flaked salmon in a big bowl.

Drizzle the salad with the citrus-mint dressing and gently toss to mix.

Serve the salad right away by dividing it into bowls.

Cassava "Rice" Bowl with Ginger-Glazed Duck

(per serving)

Serving Size: 1 bowl

Calories: 560

Fats: 34g

Carbs: 38g

Protein: 28g

Sugars: 5g

Gluten-Free: Yes

Dairy-Free: Yes

Vegan: No

For the Cassava Rice:

2 cups cassava, peeled and riced (or processed into rice-sized pieces)

1 tablespoon olive oil

Salt, to taste

For the Ginger-Glazed Duck:

2 duck breasts

1 tablespoon fresh ginger, grated

2 tablespoons coconut aminos

1 tablespoon honey (optional, adjust to taste)

Salt and pepper, to taste

For the Wilted Greens:

2 cups leafy greens (e.g. spinach, kale, or Swiss chard)

1 tablespoon olive oil

Salt, to taste

Make criss cross marks on the duck breasts' skin. Add salt and pepper for seasoning.

A skillet should be heated to medium heat. Cook the duck breasts in the skillet, skin-side down, for 6 to 8 minutes, or until the skin is golden brown and crispy.

After flipping, cook for a further 4–6 minutes, or until the internal temperature of the duck breasts reaches 165°F (74°C). After taking it out of the pan, give it some time to rest.

Remove extra grease from the same skillet, leaving roughly 1 tablespoon. Sauté the grated ginger for one minute till it becomes

aromatic. Stir together the honey (if using) and coconut aminos. Cook until slightly thickened, 2 to 3 minutes. After slicing the duck breasts, cover them with the ginger glaze.

Heat 1 tablespoon of olive oil in a separate skillet over medium heat. Season with salt and add the riced cassava. Cook, stirring occasionally, until soft and well cooked, approximately 5 to 7 minutes.

Heat 1 tablespoon of olive oil in a separate skillet over medium heat. Add a dash of salt and the leafy leaves. Sauté until wilted, approximately 2 to 3 minutes.

Layer the cassava rice, sliced duck with ginger sauce, and wilted greens in a serving dish. Over the top, drizzle any leftover ginger glaze..

Taro Root Noodle Bowl with Bone Broth

(per serving)

Serving Size: 1 bowl (approximately 2 cups)

Calories: 350

Fats: 15g

Carbs: 36g

Protein: 20g

Sugars: 3g

Gluten-Free: Yes

Dairy-Free: Yes

Paleo-Friendly: Yes

Vegan: No

2 medium taro roots (about 1 pound), spiralized

4 cups bone broth (homemade or store-bought, AIP-compliant)

8 ounces grass-fed beef, thinly sliced

1 tablespoon coconut oil

1 teaspoon fresh ginger, grated

1 clove garlic, minced (optional for AIP stage)

Salt and pepper to taste (use Himalayan salt if following AIP)

Fresh herbs for garnish (cilantro or basil)

To make Taro Noodles, first peel the taro root and use a spiralizer to turn it into strands that resemble noodles. Put aside.

Heat the coconut oil in a big saucepan or skillet over medium-high heat. Cook the grass-fed beef slices for three to five minutes, or until they are browned. Add the garlic in the last minute of cooking if using.

Add the grated ginger and the bone broth. Heat to a low simmer.

Taro noodles should be cooked by adding them to the saucepan and simmering them for a further five to seven minutes, or until the taro is soft.

As necessary, add salt and pepper to the soup after tasting it.

Transfer the bowl of noodles onto serving dishes, garnish with fresh herbs, and start eating right away..

Plantain Tortilla Wraps

(per serving)

Serving Size: 2 wraps

Calories: 350

Fats: 15g

Carbs: 40g

Protein: 20g

Sugars: 6g

Gluten-Free: Yes

Dairy-Free: Yes

Vegan: No (contains turkey)

For the Plantain Tortilla Wraps:

2 ripe plantains (yellow with some black spots)

1 tablespoon coconut oil (melted)

1/4 teaspoon sea salt

1/4 teaspoon garlic powder (optional)

For the Herb-Roasted Turkey:

1 pound turkey breast (boneless and skinless)

2 tablespoons olive oil

1 tablespoon fresh rosemary, chopped

1 tablespoon fresh thyme, chopped

1 teaspoon sea salt

1/2 teaspoon black pepper (optional)

1 tablespoon lemon juice

In order to prepare the herb-roasted turkey, first preheat the oven. Set the oven temperature to 375°F, or 190°C.

Combine the lemon juice, sea salt, rosemary, thyme, olive oil, and black pepper (if using) in a bowl. All over the turkey breast, rub this mixture.

Roast the turkey: Put the turkey in a baking dish and roast it for 25 to 30 minutes, or until it reaches 165°F (74°C) on the inside. Before slicing, let it take ten minutes to rest

Peel and chop the plantains into pieces to make the Plantain Tortilla Wraps.

Put the plantains, sea salt, melted coconut oil, and garlic powder (if using) in a food processor or blender. Blend till creamy and smooth.

A non-stick skillet should be heated to medium heat. Spread the plantain mixture in a circular shape that is approximately 1/4 inch thick after adding about 1/4 cup of it to the pan. Cook until cooked through and golden brown, approximately 2 to 3 minutes each side. Continue using the leftover mixture.

Cut the cooked turkey breast into slices.

Top each plantain tortilla with a piece of turkey and, if you'd like, some avocado or fresh greens. To make wraps, roll up the tortillas..

Sweet Potato Glass Noodle Bowl

(per serving)

Serving Size: 1 bowl

Calories: 400

Fats: 14g

Carbs: 52g

Protein: 24g

Sugars: 4g

Gluten-Free: Yes

Dairy-Free: Yes

Vegan: No (contains fish)

8 oz sweet potato glass noodles

12 oz wild-caught cod filet

2 cups bok choy, chopped

2 tablespoons coconut aminos

1 tablespoon olive oil

1 teaspoon fresh ginger, grated

1 teaspoon garlic, minced (optional, omit for strict AIP)

Salt and pepper to taste

Lime wedges for serving

Prepare the noodles by: Heat water in a saucepan until it boils. Cook the sweet potato glass noodles as directed on the box, which is typically between four and six minutes. To end cooking, drain and rinse with cold water. Put aside.

Heat the olive oil in a pan over medium heat while the noodles are cooking.

Use salt and pepper to season the cod filet. Fish should flake readily with a fork after 3–4 minutes on each side of the cod after adding it to the pan. Take out and place aside from the skillet.

Add the minced garlic (if using) and grated ginger to the same pan and cook for approximately 30 seconds, or until fragrant.

Add the coconut aminos and sliced bok choy. Sauté until wilted but still bright green, approximately 2 to 3 minutes.

Put a portion of the sweet potato glass noodles in a bowl. Place the cooked cod and the sautéed bok choy on top. If desired, drizzle with more coconut aminos.

To add a burst of flavor, serve with lime wedges on the side..

Yuca Mash Bowl with Maple-Glazed Wild Boar

(per serving)

Serving Size: 1 bowl

Calories: 550

Fats: 30g

Carbs: 50g

Protein: 30g

Sugars: 8g

Gluten-Free: Yes

Dairy-Free: Yes

Vegan: No (due to wild boar))

For the Yuca Mash:

2 cups yuca (cassava), peeled and diced

1/4 cup coconut milk

2 tablespoons olive oil

Salt (to taste)

For the Maple-Glazed Wild Boar:

1 pound wild boar, cubed

2 tablespoons olive oil

2 tablespoons pure maple syrup

1 teaspoon garlic powder

1 teaspoon onion powder

Salt and pepper (to taste)

For the Caramelized Vegetables:

1 cup carrots, sliced

1 cup bell peppers, sliced

1 cup onions, sliced

2 tablespoons olive oil

Salt (to taste)

Bring a big saucepan of water that has been salted to a boil.

Add the diced yuca and simmer until it's soft, around 20-25 minutes

Return to the pot after draining. Mash until smooth after adding the coconut milk and olive oil. Add salt to taste. Put aside.

Put two teaspoons of olive oil in a pan over medium heat.

Season with salt, pepper, onion powder, garlic powder, and diced wild boar. Cook for about 5-7 minutes or until browned.

Add maple syrup and heat for an additional 3–4 minutes until cooked through and glazed. Put aside.

Put two tablespoons of olive oil in the same skillet. Add the bell peppers, onions, and carrot slices. The veggies should be soft and caramelized after around 10-15 minutes of sautéing over medium heat, stirring periodically. Add salt to taste.

In a dish, arrange the maple-glazed wild boar, a large portion of caramelized veggies, and a layer of creamy yuca mash.

Coconut "Rice" Bowl with Lemongrass Chicken

(per serving)

Serving Size: 1 bowl

Calories: 400

Fats: 25g

Carbs: 25g

Protein: 25g

Sugars: 2g

Gluten-Free: Yes

Dairy-Free: Yes

Vegan: No (contains chicken)

For the Coconut Rice:

2 cups riced coconut meat (fresh or frozen)

1 cup coconut milk (unsweetened)

1/2 teaspoon sea salt

1 tablespoon lime juice

For the Lemongrass Chicken:

1 lb chicken breast, thinly sliced

2 stalks lemongrass, minced

2 cloves garlic, minced

1 tablespoon fresh ginger, minced

2 tablespoons coconut aminos (AIP-friendly soy sauce substitute)

2 tablespoons coconut oil

Fresh herbs for garnish (such as cilantro or basil)

First, make the coconut rice: Put the riced coconut flesh, coconut milk, sea salt, and lime juice in a medium pot. Cook over medium heat for 5 to 7 minutes, stirring periodically, until cooked through and well mixed. Take off the heat and put it aside.

Add the sliced chicken, coconut aminos, ginger, garlic, and chopped lemongrass to a bowl. After thoroughly coating the chicken, let it marinade for about fifteen minutes.

Heat the coconut oil in a big pan over medium-high heat. Add the marinated chicken and heat, moving periodically, until golden brown and cooked through, 5 to 7 minutes.

The coconut rice should be divided among serving dishes.

Place the lemongrass chicken on top and add some fresh herbs as a garnish.

Serve right away.

Japanese-Style Kelp Noodle Bowl

(per serving)

Serving Size: 1 bowl (recipe serves 2)

Calories: 290

Fats: 14g

Carbs: 13g

Protein: 28g

Sugars: 2g

Gluten-Free: Yes

Dairy-Free: Yes

Low-Carb: Yes

Paleo: Yes

Vegan: No (due to scallops)

8 oz kelp noodles (rinsed and drained)

1 lb scallops (fresh, patted dry)

2 tablespoons olive oil (or avocado oil)

1 tablespoon coconut aminos

1 teaspoon fresh ginger, grated

1 tablespoon lime juice

1 cup bok choy or spinach (chopped)

1 green onion (sliced, for garnish)

Sesame seeds (optional, for garnish)

After giving the kelp noodles a quick rinse in cold water, put them aside. To make them even softer, you may soak them in warm water for ten minutes or so.

Heat 1 tablespoon of olive oil in a pan over medium heat. Sauté the spinach or bok choy for two to three minutes, or until they wilt. Take out and place aside from the skillet.

Put an additional tablespoon of olive oil in the same skillet.

Heat until it shimmers over medium-high heat.

Add a dash of salt and pepper to the scallops (don't add pepper if you're following strict AIP).

Make sure the scallops are not packed too tightly in the skillet. Sear until cooked through and golden brown, 2 to 3 minutes each side. Take off the heat.

Add the grated ginger, coconut aminos, lime juice, sautéed greens, and kelp noodles to a bowl. Gently toss to combine.

Place the cooked scallops on top of the noodle mixture. If used, garnish with sesame seeds and chopped green onion. Have fun!.

Roasted Spaghetti Squash

(per serving)

Serving Size: 1/2 squash with sauce (approximately 1.5 cups total)

Calories: 220

Fats: 9g

Carbs: 34g

Protein: 5g

Sugars: 5g

Gluten-Free: Yes

Dairy-Free: Yes

Vegan: Yes

AIP-Friendly: Yes (if black pepper is omitted)

1 medium spaghetti squash

2 tablespoons olive oil

1 teaspoon sea salt

1/2 teaspoon black pepper (omit if strictly AIP)

2 cups wild mushrooms (shiitake, oyster, or porcini), sliced

2 cloves garlic, minced

1 small onion, diced

1 tablespoon fresh thyme leaves (or 1 teaspoon dried thyme)

1 tablespoon coconut aminos (for a touch of sweetness)

1 cup vegetable broth (low sodium, if needed)

1 tablespoon apple cider vinegar (for brightness)

The first step is to preheat the oven to 400°F (200°C).

Cut the spaghetti squash lengthwise in half, then scoop out the seeds.

Sprinkle with half a teaspoon of salt and pepper (if using) and drizzle with one tablespoon of olive oil.

Arrange the squash cut-side down on a parchment paper-lined baking sheet.

The meat should be tender and penetrated with a fork after 30 to 40 minutes of roasting in a preheated oven.

The third step is to prepare the mushroom sauce: Heat the remaining tablespoon of olive oil in a large pan over medium heat while the squash roasts.

Sauté the chopped onion for three to four minutes, or until it becomes transparent.

After adding the sliced mushrooms and minced garlic, simmer for an additional five to seven minutes, or until the mushrooms are soft and browned.

Cook for a further minute after adding the coconut aminos and thyme.

Bring the mixture to a simmer after adding the apple cider vinegar and vegetable broth. Allow the sauce to thicken a little by cooking it for five to seven minutes.

After the spaghetti squash is cooked, take it out of the oven and allow it to cool for a few minutes before serving.

Scrape the meat into strands that resemble noodles with a fork.

Serve the wild mushroom sauce over the spaghetti squash noodles..

Braised Duck Legs with Caramelized Apples

(per serving)

Serving Size: 1 duck leg with apples

Calories: 450

Fats: 30g

Carbs: 20g

Protein: 30g

Sugars: 10g (naturally occurring from apples and honey)

Gluten-Free: Yes

Dairy-Free: Yes

AIP: Yes (omit black pepper and honey for strict AIP))

4 duck legs

1 tablespoon coconut oil

1 teaspoon sea salt (adjust to taste)

1/2 teaspoon black pepper (omit for strict AIP)

2 cups low-sodium chicken or vegetable broth

2 tablespoons apple cider vinegar

3 medium sweet-tart apples (like Honeycrisp or Granny Smith), cored and sliced

1 teaspoon cinnamon

1 tablespoon honey (optional, adjust to taste)

First, sear the duck legs: Heat the coconut oil in a large Dutch oven or heavy-bottomed pot over medium-high heat.

Use sea salt and black pepper (if using) to season the duck legs. After putting the duck legs in the pot skin-side down, sear them for five to seven minutes, or until the skin is golden brown. For a further five minutes, flip and sear the other side.

Take out and reserve the duck legs. Leave roughly 1 tablespoon of fat in the saucepan after draining the excess.

While scraping off any browned pieces from the bottom of the saucepan, add the apple cider vinegar and broth.

Skin-side up, put the duck legs back in the saucepan. Reduce the heat to low, cover, and bring to a simmer. The duck should be cooked for

one and a half to two hours, or until it is soft and separates from the bone easily.

Add the cinnamon and sliced apples to the pot around half an hour before the duck is done. Drizzle honey over apples if using. Gently stir to mix.

Continue cooking with the lid back on until the apples are soft and have caramelized.

Take the duck legs out of the saucepan and let them rest for a few minutes. Drizzle the cooking liquid over the duck legs and garnish with the caramelized apples.

Poached Cod in Ginger-Turmeric Broth

(per serving)

Serving Size: 1 cod filet with broth

Calories: 230

Fats: 9g

Carbs: 7g

Protein: 30g

Sugars: 1g

Gluten-Free: Yes

Dairy-Free: Yes

Vegan: No (fish is used)

4 (6 oz) cod filets (fresh or thawed)

2 cups vegetable broth (low-sodium, AIP-compliant)

1 tablespoon fresh ginger, grated

1 teaspoon ground turmeric

1 tablespoon coconut aminos

1 clove garlic, minced (optional for AIP)

1 tablespoon olive oil (for serving)

Salt and pepper to taste (optional for AIP)

Fresh cilantro or parsley for garnish

Put the vegetable broth, ground turmeric, grated ginger, coconut aminos, and chopped garlic (if using) in a big pot. On medium heat, bring to a moderate simmer.

Carefully dip the fish filets into the boiling liquid. The fish should be opaque and flake readily with a fork after 10 to 12 minutes of poaching, covered in the pan.

Spoon the poached fish onto plates using a slotted spoon. Over the fish, ladle the ginger-turmeric broth. Garnish with parsley or fresh cilantro and drizzle with olive oil.

Warm up and savor the filling tastes.

Roasted Bone Marrow with Herb-Infused Parsnip Puree

(per serving, serves 2)

Serving Size: 2 marrow bones with parsnip puree

Calories: 480

Fats: 38g

Carbs: 25g

Protein: 16g

Sugars: 6g

Gluten-Free: Yes

Dairy-Free: Yes

Vegan: No (contains animal products)

For the Roasted Bone Marrow:

4 large marrow bones (about 6-8 inches long, cut in half)

Salt (to taste)

Fresh herbs for garnish (such as parsley or thyme)

For the Herb-Infused Parsnip Puree:

2 large parsnips, peeled and chopped

1 tablespoon olive oil

1 cup vegetable broth (homemade or low-sodium)

1 teaspoon fresh thyme or other AIP-friendly herbs

Salt and pepper (to taste)

Set the oven's temperature to 450°F, or 230°C.

To roast the bone marrow, arrange the bones on a baking sheet in an upright position. Add salt for seasoning.

The marrow should be tender and bubbling after 15 to 20 minutes of roasting in a preheated oven.

Take it out of the oven and let it cool a little.

Heat the olive oil in a saucepan over medium heat while the marrow roasts.

After adding the chopped parsnips, cook for about five minutes.

Bring to a simmer after adding the veggie broth. Cook for 15 to 20 minutes, or until the parsnips are soft.

Season with salt and pepper to taste and add the thyme.

Puree the contents in a blender until it's smooth.

Form a bed for the roasted marrow bones by spooning the parsnip puree onto plates.

Place the heated marrow on top of the parsnip puree after scooping it out of the bones.

Before serving, garnish with fresh herbs..

Steamed Mussels in Lemongrass-Coconut Broth

(per serving, assuming 4 servings)

Serving Size: Approximately ½ lb mussels with broth

Calories: 220

Fats: 12g

Carbs: 10g

Protein: 20g

Sugars: 2g

Gluten-Free: Yes

Dairy-Free: Yes

Vegan: No (due to mussels)

2 lbs fresh mussels, cleaned and debearded

1 can (14 oz) coconut milk (full fat)

1 stalk lemongrass, trimmed and smashed

2 cups vegetable broth (low sodium)

1-inch piece of fresh ginger, sliced

2 cloves garlic, minced

1 tablespoon fish sauce (optional, adjust for AIP)

Juice of 1 lime

Fresh cilantro leaves for garnish

Red chili flakes or sliced fresh chili (optional, for heat)

Put the coconut milk, vegetable broth, sliced ginger, chopped garlic, crushed lemongrass, and fish sauce (if using) in a big saucepan. Bring over medium heat to a simmer.

Put the cleaned mussels into the saucepan when the liquid has begun to boil. The mussels should open after 5 to 7 minutes of steaming under cover. Any mussels that stay unopened should be thrown out.

Turn off the heat when the mussels are done. Add the lime juice and taste to adjust the seasoning.

Top the mussels with the flavorful broth and sprinkle with fresh cilantro before serving them in bowls. If desired, add fresh chili or red chili flakes for heat.

Pan-Seared Rabbit with Roasted Root Vegetables

(per serving, assuming 2 servings)

Serving Size: 1 rabbit leg with vegetables

Calories: 350

Fats: 15g

Carbs: 30g

Protein: 35g

Sugars: 8g

Gluten-Free: Yes

Dairy-Free: Yes

AIP-Friendly: Yes

2 rabbit legs or whole rabbit, cut into pieces

2 tablespoons olive oil or coconut oil

1 teaspoon fresh rosemary, chopped or ½ teaspoon dried rosemary

1 teaspoon fresh thyme, chopped or ½ teaspoon dried thyme

Salt (to taste)

Black pepper (optional; omit for strict AIP)

1 cup carrots, chopped

1 cup sweet potatoes, diced

1 cup parsnips, diced

1 cup turnips, diced

1 tablespoon fresh lemon juice

The first step is to preheat the oven to 400°F (200°C).

Combine 1 tablespoon of olive oil, salt, rosemary, thyme, and sliced carrots, sweet potatoes, parsnips, and turnips in a big bowl.

Arrange the veggies in a single layer on a baking sheet.

The vegetables should be roasted in a warm oven for around 25-30 minutes, or until they are soft and have a hint of caramel. To ensure consistent cooking, toss halfway through.

In a large pan over medium-high heat, heat 1 tablespoon of olive oil while the veggies roast.

Use salt and black pepper (if using) to season the rabbit pieces.

When the rabbit is golden brown and cooked through, add it to the skillet and sear it for 5–6 minutes on each side. A temperature of 160°F (71°C) should be reached within.

The rabbit should be served with the roasted root vegetables after being drizzled with lemon juice..

Wild-Caught Sardines with Fennel-Apple Slaw

(per serving, using canned sardines)

Serving Size: 1 can sardines with slaw

Calories: 310

Fats: 20g

Carbs: 14g

Protein: 24g

Sugars: 6g

Gluten-Free: Yes

Dairy-Free: Yes

Vegan: No (due to sardines))

For the Sardines:

2 cans (4 oz each) wild-caught sardines in olive oil (or fresh sardines, if preferred)

1 tablespoon olive oil (if using fresh sardines)

Salt (to taste)

Pepper (optional, omit for AIP)

For the Fennel-Apple Slaw:

1 cup fennel bulb, thinly sliced

1 cup green apple, julienned (such as Granny Smith)

1 tablespoon fresh lemon juice

1 tablespoon apple cider vinegar

1 tablespoon extra virgin olive oil

Salt (to taste)

1 tablespoon fresh dill or parsley (optional, for garnish)

Place the julienned apple and sliced fennel in a basin.

Whisk the lemon juice, apple cider vinegar, olive oil, and salt in a separate small bowl.

Toss the apple and fennel combination with the dressing after adding it. Give it twenty minutes or so to develop flavors and soften a little.

Heat olive oil in a pan over medium heat if using fresh sardines.

Add salt (and pepper, if using) and fry the sardines for 3–4 minutes on each side, or until they are golden brown and cooked through.

Just drain and reheat the tinned sardines in the pan for two to three minutes.

Arrange the fennel-apple slaw over the fried sardines on a dish.

If desired, garnish with parsley or fresh dill. Serve right away..

Dinners for Rest and Recovery

Ginger-Turmeric Poached Cod with Wilted Greens

(per serving)

Serving Size: 1 cod filet with wilted greens

Calories: 350

Fats: 20g

Carbs: 12g

Protein: 30g

Sugars: 2g

Gluten-Free: Yes

Dairy-Free: Yes

Vegan: No

For the Poached Cod:

2 cod filets (about 6 oz each)

1 can (13.5 oz) coconut milk

1 tablespoon fresh ginger, grated

1 tablespoon fresh turmeric, grated or 1 teaspoon turmeric powder

1 tablespoon fresh herbs (parsley or cilantro)

Salt, to taste (optional)

For the Wilted Greens:

4 cups collard greens, chopped

2 cloves garlic, minced

1 tablespoon olive oil (optional)

Salt, to taste (optional)

Put the coconut milk, grated ginger, grated turmeric, and herbs in a medium pot. Heat over medium-low until heated, stirring well.

Make sure the cod filets are completely immersed in the coconut milk mixture after adding them to the pot. The fish should flake readily with a fork after 10 to 12 minutes of simmering under cover.

In a large skillet over medium heat, heat the olive oil (if using) while the cod poaches. Sauté the minced garlic for one to two minutes, or until it becomes aromatic.

Toss the chopped collard greens with the garlic in the pan. Cook until soft and wilted, approximately 3 to 5 minutes. If desired, add salt for seasoning.

Put the poached fish on a dish with the wilted collard greens. Drizzle the fish and greens with a spoonful of the ginger-turmeric coconut milk sauce..

Wild Salmon and Fennel En Papillote

(per serving)

Serving Size: 1 salmon filet with fennel

Calories: 300

Fats: 18g

Carbs: 6g

Protein: 28g

Sugars: 1g

Gluten-Free: Yes

Dairy-Free: Yes

Vegan: No (contains fish)

2 wild-caught salmon filets (about 6 ounces each)

1 medium bulb of fennel, thinly sliced

2 tablespoons fresh dill, chopped or other herbs like parsley or thyme

1 tablespoon olive oil

Juice of 1 lemon

Salt and pepper to taste (omit pepper for strict AIP)

Set the oven temperature to 400°F (200°C).

Cut two big (12 x 16 inch) pieces of parchment paper.

Lay sliced fennel on one side of each sheet of paper. Place a salmon filet on top. Drizzle with olive oil, pour lemon juice over the top, and sprinkle with fresh dill. If used, season with salt.

Fourth, seal the packets: Over the salmon and fennel, fold the other side of the paper. Tightly seal the package by making tiny overlapping folds beginning at one end, leaving a little opening for steam to flow through.

The salmon should be cooked through and flake easily with a fork after placing the packets on a baking sheet and baking them in a preheated oven for about 15–20 minutes.

Carefully open the packets (be mindful of steam!) and serve right away, covering the salmon and fennel with any juices..

Sardine-Stuffed Avocado Boats

(per serving)

Serving Size: 1 avocado half stuffed with sardines

Calories: 330

Fats: 27g

Carbs: 13g

Protein: 10g

Sugars: 1g

Gluten-Free: Yes

Dairy-Free: Yes

Vegan: No (contains sardines)

2 fresh sardines, cleaned and fileted

1 tablespoon olive oil

1 tablespoon fresh parsley, chopped

1 tablespoon fresh dill, chopped

Juice of 1/2 lemon

Salt, to taste (optional)

1 ripe avocado, halved and pitted

Microgreens, for garnish

Put the sardine filets, olive oil, lemon juice, parsley, dill, and salt in a basin. Make sure the sardines are well covered with the oil and herbs by gently mixing them together.

The second step is to stuff avocados. Put the avocado halves on a dish. Load each avocado half with a spoonful of the sardine mixture.

Add microgreens on top for extra nutrition and taste.

Mediterranean-Style Mackerel with Herbs

(per serving)

Serving Size: 1 mackerel filet with vegetables

Calories: 400

Fats: 28g

Carbs: 15g

Protein: 30g

Sugars: 6g

Gluten-Free: Yes

Dairy-Free: Yes

AIP-Friendly: Yes (omit pepper)

For the Mackerel:

2 mackerel filets (fresh or thawed)

2 tablespoons olive oil

2 tablespoons fresh parsley, chopped

2 tablespoons fresh basil, chopped

1 tablespoon fresh oregano, chopped

2 cloves garlic, minced

Juice of 1 lemon

Salt and pepper, to taste (omit pepper for strict AIP)

For the Roasted Mediterranean Vegetables:

1 zucchini, sliced

1 bell pepper (any color), chopped

1 small red onion, chopped

1 cup cherry tomatoes, halved

2 tablespoons olive oil

1 teaspoon dried oregano

Salt and pepper, to taste (omit pepper for strict AIP)

The first step is to preheat the oven to 400°F (200°C).

Combine the bell pepper, red onion, cherry tomatoes, and zucchini in a large bowl.

Season with salt (and pepper, if using), add dried oregano, and drizzle with olive oil. Toss to ensure even coating.

Arrange the veggies in a single layer on a baking sheet.

Roast in a preheated oven for 20 to 25 minutes, tossing halfway through, or until soft and beginning to caramelize.

Heat the olive oil in a pan over medium-high heat while the veggies roast.

After patting the mackerel filets dry, season them with salt and, if desired, pepper.

Skin-side down, place the mackerel in the skillet. Cook until the fish is cooked through and flakes easily with a fork, about 4–5 minutes. Carefully turn and cook for another 3–4 minutes.

To give the fish more flavor in the last minute of cooking, add half a lemon and chopped garlic to the pan with the mackerel.

Arrange the pan-seared mackerel on top of the roasted Mediterranean vegetables on a plate. Before serving, sprinkle with fresh herbs and drizzle with more lemon juice.

.

Herb-Crusted Arctic Char

(per serving)

Serving Size: 1 Arctic char filet with roasted vegetables

Calories: 360

Fats: 18g

Carbs: 35g

Protein: 24g

Sugars: 8g

Gluten-Free: Yes

Dairy-Free: Yes

Vegan: No

For the Herb-Crusted Arctic Char:

2 Arctic char filets (about 6 oz each)

2 tablespoons olive oil

1/4 cup fresh parsley, chopped

1/4 cup fresh dill, chopped

1 teaspoon garlic powder

Salt and pepper to taste (omit pepper for strict AIP)

For the Roasted Root Vegetables:

2 medium sweet potatoes, diced

2 medium carrots, sliced

1 parsnip, diced

2 tablespoons olive oil

Salt and herbs of choice (e.g. thyme or rosemary)

The first step is to preheat the oven to 400°F (200°C).

Diced sweet potatoes, carrots, and parsnips should be combined with salt, herbs, and 2 tablespoons of olive oil in a big bowl.

Arrange the veggies in a single layer on a parchment paper-lined baking sheet.

Third, roast the vegetables in a warm oven for 25 to 30 minutes, stirring halfway through, or until they are soft and gently browned.

In a separate bowl, combine the chopped parsley, dill, garlic powder, and 2 tablespoons olive oil while the veggies roast. Your herb crust will look like this.

Arrange the filets of Arctic char on a parchment paper-lined baking dish. Gently massage the herb combination and salt onto the fish to season it.

Place the baking dish with the herb-crusted Arctic char in the oven after the veggies have been roasting for about fifteen minutes.

Bake for another 12 to 15 minutes, or until the fish is cooked through and flakes readily with a fork.

Present the roasted root vegetables with the herb-crusted Arctic char..

Saffron-Infused Mussels

(per serving, based on 4 servings)

Serving Size: Approximately 1/2 pound mussels with broth

Calories: 210

Fats: 8g

Carbs: 6g

Protein: 26g

Sugars: 1g

2 pounds fresh mussels, cleaned and debearded

2 cups bone broth (chicken or vegetable, homemade is best)

1/4 teaspoon saffron threads

2 tablespoons olive oil

4 cloves garlic, minced

1 teaspoon fresh thyme leaves (or 1/2 teaspoon dried thyme)

1 teaspoon fresh oregano leaves (or 1/2 teaspoon dried oregano)

Salt and pepper to taste

1/4 cup fresh parsley, chopped (for garnish)

Gluten-Free: Yes

Dairy-Free: Yes

Vegan: No

Heat the bone broth in a pot over medium heat. To release the taste and color, add the saffron threads and soak for about five minutes.

Heat the olive oil in a big saucepan over a medium heat. Be cautious not to burn the minced garlic when you add it and sauté it for one to two minutes until fragrant.

Cook for one more minute after adding the oregano and thyme.

Pour the bone broth with saffron into the saucepan after adding the cleaned mussels. The mussels should open after 5 to 7 minutes of steaming in a covered saucepan. Any mussels that don't open should be thrown away.

Add salt and pepper to taste and adjust the broth.

Season with fresh parsley and serve by ladling the mussels and liquid into dishes.

Pan-Seared Halibut with Citrus

(per serving)

Serving Size: 1 halibut filet with roasted fennel

Calories: 350

Fats: 20g

Carbs: 12g

Protein: 36g

Sugars: 3g

Gluten-Free: Yes

Dairy-Free: Yes

Vegan: No

2 (6-ounce) halibut filets

1 tablespoon olive oil (or avocado oil)

Zest of 1 orange

Zest of 1 lemon

Salt (to taste, optional)

Pepper (to taste, optional)

1 large bulb of fennel, sliced

2 tablespoons fresh herbs (such as parsley or dill), chopped

Juice of 1 lemon

The first step is to preheat the oven to 400°F (200°C).

Arrange the sliced fennel on a baking sheet with a little olive oil and a sprinkle of salt (if using). Bake for about 20-25 minutes, or until soft and beginning to caramelize.

While the fennel roasts, rub the halibut filets with salt (if using), pepper, and citrus zest.

In a large pan, heat the olive oil over medium-high heat. When the pan is heated, gently add the halibut filets. The fish should be golden brown and flake readily with a fork after approximately **4-5 minutes** of searing on each side.

For extra flavor, pour fresh lemon juice over the halibut in the last minute of cooking.

Place the pan-seared halibut on top of the roasted fennel. As a garnish, add more citrus zest and fresh herbs..

Bone Broth Braised Lamb Shanks

(per serving, based on 4 servings)

Serving Size: 1 lamb shank with vegetables

Calories: 400

Fats: 22g

Carbs: 18g

Protein: 32g

Sugars: 4g

Gluten-Free: Yes

Dairy-Free: Yes

AIP Compliant: Yes

4 lamb shanks

4 cups bone broth (homemade or store-bought, ensure it's AIP compliant)

2 tablespoons olive oil (or coconut oil)

1 large onion, chopped

3 cloves garlic, minced

2 large carrots, chopped

2 parsnips, chopped

1 medium sweet potato, chopped

1 tablespoon fresh rosemary, chopped or 1 teaspoon dried

1 tablespoon fresh thyme, chopped or 1 teaspoon dried

Salt and pepper to taste (omit or use a pinch if strictly AIP)

1 bay leaf

First, sear the lamb shanks. Heat the olive oil in a large Dutch oven or heavy saucepan over medium-high heat. If using, season the lamb shanks with salt and pepper. Then, fry them for 5 to 7 minutes on both sides, or until browned. Take out and put aside.

Add the chopped garlic and onion to the same saucepan. The onion should be transparent after two to three minutes of sautéing. Cook for a further five minutes after adding the sweet potato, carrots, and parsnips.

Scrape the bottom of the saucepan to get rid of any browned parts before adding the bone broth. Return the seared lamb shanks to the saucepan with the bay leaf, thyme, and rosemary.

Slow Cook: Lower the heat to low after bringing to a simmer. The lamb should be soft and fall off the bone after two and a half to three hours of cooking under cover. This may also be cooked for 6 to 8 hours on low in a slow cooker.

After the lamb shanks are done, take them out of the pot and give them some time to rest. If preferred, top the lamb with fresh herbs and serve it with the veggies and broth..

Herb-Stuffed Pastured Turkey Breast

(per serving, assuming 6 servings)

Serving Size: 1 slice of turkey with vegetables

Calories: 280

Fats: 12g

Carbs: 20g

Protein: 30g

Sugars: 5g

Gluten-Free: Yes

Dairy-Free: Yes

AIP-Friendly: Yes

For the Turkey:

2 lbs pastured turkey breast

1/2 cup fresh parsley, chopped

1/4 cup fresh thyme, chopped

1/4 cup fresh rosemary, chopped

2 cloves garlic, minced

1 tablespoon olive oil

Salt and pepper to taste (use salt sparingly to keep it AIP-friendly)

For the Roasted Vegetables:

2 cups carrots, chopped

2 cups zucchini, chopped

1 cup bell peppers, chopped

1 tablespoon olive oil

1 teaspoon dried oregano

Salt and pepper to taste (optional)

Set the oven's temperature to 375°F (190°C).

Combine the chopped parsley, olive oil, minced garlic, thyme, rosemary, salt, and pepper in a bowl. This will be your stuffing with herbs.

Gently cut a pocket into the breast of the bird. Gently push the herb mixture into the pocket to make sure it is evenly distributed.

Combine the diced bell peppers, zucchini, and carrots in a big bowl with the olive oil, oregano, salt, and pepper (if using). Evenly distribute them on a baking pan.

Position the filled turkey breast and the veggies in the middle of the baking sheet.

The turkey should be cooked thoroughly (internal temperature should reach 165°F or 74°C) and the veggies should be soft after 60 to 75 minutes of roasting in a preheated oven.

Before slicing, let the turkey rest for ten minutes or so. Serve with the roasted veggies.

Grass-Fed Beef Heart with Chimichurri

(per serving, serves 4)

Serving Size: 1/4 of the dish (approx. 4 oz beef heart + 1/2 cup sweet potatoes)

Calories: 300

Fats: 20g

Carbs: 25g

Protein: 18g

Sugars: 5g

Gluten-Free: Yes

Dairy-Free: Yes

Vegan: No

For the Beef Heart:

1 lb grass-fed beef heart, cleaned and sliced thinly

2 tablespoons olive oil

Salt and pepper to taste (use sea salt for AIP)

For the Chimichurri:

1 cup fresh parsley, finely chopped

1/2 cup fresh cilantro, finely chopped

3 cloves garlic, minced

1/4 cup olive oil

2 tablespoons red wine vinegar

1 teaspoon dried oregano

Salt to taste

For the Roasted Sweet Potatoes:

2 medium sweet potatoes, peeled and cut into cubes

2 tablespoons olive oil

Salt and pepper to taste (use sea salt for AIP)

1 teaspoon paprika (optional)

Add the dried oregano, olive oil, red wine vinegar, chopped parsley, cilantro, minced garlic, and salt to a bowl. To let the flavors blend, thoroughly mix and put away.

The second step is to roast the sweet potatoes: Set the oven's temperature to 400°F, or 200°C.

Add the olive oil, salt, pepper, and paprika (if using) to the cubes of sweet potato. Line a baking sheet with them.

They should be soft and golden brown after 25 to 30 minutes of roasting, rotating them halfway through.

In a pan, heat the olive oil over medium-high heat.

Add salt and pepper to the thinly sliced beef heart.

Slices of beef heart should be cooked to your preferred doneness after 3–4 minutes on each side of the pan.

Arrange the beef heart slices on a plate and cover with a good amount of chimichurri.

Serve with sweet potatoes that have been roasted.

Duck Confit with Lavender

(per serving)

Serving Size: 1 duck leg with vegetables

Calories: 570

Fats: 42g

Carbs: 30g

Protein: 30g

Sugars: 6g

Gluten-Free: Yes

Dairy-Free: Yes

AIP-Friendly: Yes (if black pepper is omitted)

4 duck legs

1 cup duck fat (or enough to submerge the duck legs)

1 tablespoon dried culinary lavender

2 cloves garlic, crushed

1 tablespoon fresh rosemary, chopped

1 tablespoon fresh thyme, chopped

Salt, to taste (preferably sea salt)

Freshly ground black pepper, to taste (optional, depending on AIP tolerance)

Roasted Root Vegetables

2 carrots, chopped

2 parsnips, chopped

1 sweet potato, chopped

1 red onion, quartered

2 tablespoons olive oil

Salt, to taste

1 teaspoon dried thyme

For the Duck Confit:

Use paper towels to pat the duck legs dry. Sprinkle them liberally with thyme, lavender, garlic, rosemary, salt, and pepper, if using. For optimal taste, let them marinade in the fridge for at least an hour or overnight.

Adjust the oven temperature to 225°F (107°C) in order to slowly cook the duck. Place the duck legs in a large saucepan or Dutch oven and pour duck grease over them. Make sure the legs are fully immersed.

Cover and cook for about 4–5 hours in a preheated oven, or until the flesh is soft and separates from the bone easily.

Take the duck legs out of the fat and put them on a baking sheet, skin side up, if you want crispy skin. Watch carefully to avoid burning while you broil for three to five minutes.

In order to prepare the roasted root vegetables, first preheat the oven to 400°F (200°C).

Combine the chopped red onion, sweet potato, parsnips, and carrots with olive oil, salt, and dried thyme in a big basin.

Arrange the veggies in a single layer on a baking sheet. Stir halfway through and roast for 25 to 30 minutes, or until golden brown and soft.

Present a big amount of roasted root vegetables on a platter with the duck confit. If desired, drizzle with some of the duck fat..

Rosemary-Infused Venison Medallions

(per serving, based on 4 servings)

Serving Size: 1 medallion with mashed celery root

Calories: 350

Fats: 20g

Carbs: 15g

Protein: 30g

Sugars: 2g

Gluten-Free: Yes

Dairy-Free: Yes

AIP-Friendly: Yes

For the Venison Medallions:

1 lb venison loin, cut into medallions

2 tablespoons olive oil or avocado oil for AIP

2-3 sprigs fresh rosemary, leaves stripped

Salt and pepper to taste (use salt if AIP allows)

For the Mashed Celery Root:

1 medium celery root (celeriac), peeled and diced

1/4 cup coconut milk (or more for desired creaminess)

2 tablespoons olive oil (or avocado oil)

Salt to taste (optional)

Fresh chives or parsley for garnish (optional)

Bring salted water to a boil in a kettle. Cook for approximately 20 minutes after adding the chopped celery root until it becomes soft. Return to the pot after draining. Mash until smooth after adding the coconut milk and olive oil. If required, add more salt to adjust the seasoning. Put aside.

In a pan, heat the olive oil over medium-high heat.

Use salt and pepper to season the venison medallions. Add the venison medallions to the pan with the heated oil.

The medallions should be browned and cooked to your preferred doneness after 3–4 minutes on each side of the grill (medium-rare is usually advised for venison).

Add the fresh rosemary to the pan and let it absorb the meat and oil in the last minute of cooking.

Arrange the venison medallions flavored with rosemary on top of the mashed celery root. If desired, garnish with chopped parsley or chives.

Slow-Cooked Oxtail with Ginger

(per serving)

Serving Size: About 1/2 lb of oxtail and 1/2 cup of carrots

Calories: 420

Fats: 28g

Carbs: 15g

Protein: 32g

Sugars: 4g

Gluten-Free: Yes

Dairy-Free: Yes

Vegan: No

2 lbs oxtail, cut into pieces

1 tablespoon coconut oil

1 large onion, diced

4 cloves garlic, minced

2 tablespoons fresh ginger, grated

4 cups bone broth (beef or vegetable)

2 carrots, chopped

1 tablespoon fresh thyme leaves

1 tablespoon fresh rosemary, chopped

Salt (to taste, optional)

Pepper (to taste, optional)

Heat the coconut oil in a big pan over medium-high heat. If using, season the oxtail with salt and pepper. Sear the chunks for 5 to 7 minutes, or until browned on both sides. Put in a slow cooker.

Add the chopped onion to the same pan and cook for about five minutes, or until it is tender. Cook the ginger and garlic for a further two minutes, or until fragrant.

Cover the oxtail in the slow cooker with the onion mixture. Add sliced carrots, rosemary, thyme, and bone broth. Mix to blend.

The oxtail should be soft and fall from the bone after 8 to 10 hours of cooking on low, covered.

When the oxtail is done, take it out of the slow cooker. Serve the roasted carrots and some of the broth beside the oxtail.

For the roasted carrots, you can simply toss sliced carrots with a bit of coconut oil and sea salt, then roast them in the oven at 400°F (200°C) for 25-30 minutes until tender and slightly caramelized.

Roasted Kabocha Squash with Sage

(per serving)

Serving Size: 1 cup of roasted kabocha squash

Calories: 160

Fats: 7g

Carbs: 23g

Protein: 2g

Sugars: 4g

Gluten-Free: Yes

Dairy-Free: Yes

Vegan: Yes

1 medium kabocha squash

2 tablespoons olive oil

1 teaspoon sea salt (adjust to taste)

1 tablespoon fresh sage leaves (chopped or whole)

The first step is to preheat the oven to 400°F (200°C).

Split the kabocha squash in two and remove the seeds with a spoon. The skin is edible and nutrient-dense, but you may peel it if you'd like.

Depending on your taste, cut the squash into cubes or wedges.

Toss the squash in a big bowl with sea salt, olive oil, and fresh sage until it's covered evenly.

Line a baking sheet with parchment paper and spread the squash in a single layer. Roast, turning halfway through, in a preheated oven for 25 to 30 minutes, or until the squash is soft and caramelized.

To serve, take it out of the oven and allow it to cool a little..

Watermelon Radish Carpaccio

(per serving)

Serving Size: 1 cup of sliced radishes (about 4 servings total)

Calories: 50

Fats: 5g

Carbs: 6g

Protein: 1g

Sugars: 2g

Gluten-Free: Yes

Dairy-Free: Yes

Vegan: Yes)

2 medium watermelon radishes (thinly sliced)

2 tablespoons extra virgin olive oil

1 tablespoon fresh lemon juice

1 tablespoon fresh herbs (basil, parsley, or cilantro), finely chopped

Sea salt (to taste)

Freshly cracked black pepper (optional, omit for strict AIP)

Microgreens or additional herbs for garnish (optional)

Lightly slice the watermelon radishes with a sharp knife or a mandoline slicer, then place them in a single layer on a serving tray.

Whisk the lemon juice, sea salt, chopped herbs, and olive oil in a small dish. Taste and adjust the seasoning.

Evenly drizzle the sliced radishes with the dressing.

If preferred, garnish with more herbs or microgreens. Serve right away as a cool side dish or appetizer.

.

Roasted Purple Sweet Potato with Rosemary

(per serving)

Serving Size: About 1 cup of roasted wedges

Calories: 180

Fats: 8g

Carbs: 30g

Protein: 2g

Sugars: 7g

Gluten-Free: Yes

Dairy-Free: Yes

Vegan: Yes

2 medium purple sweet potatoes

2 tablespoons olive oil

2 tablespoons fresh rosemary, chopped

Salt to taste (optional, use a salt substitute if strictly AIP)

The first step is to preheat the oven to 400°F (200°C).

Clean the purple sweet potatoes and peel them. Slice them into cubes or wedges that are about an inch thick.

Combine the sweet potato wedges, chopped rosemary, olive oil, and a bit of salt (if using) in a big dish.

Line a baking sheet with parchment paper and spread the seasoned sweet potatoes in a single layer.

Preheat the oven for 25 to 30 minutes. Turn the sweet potatoes halfway through, or until they are soft and just beginning to turn brown.

To serve, take it out of the oven and allow it to cool a little..

Caramelized Fennel and Artichoke Hearts

(per serving)

Serving Size: About 1 cup

Calories: 150

Fats: 11g

Carbs: 13g

Protein: 2g

Sugars: 3g

Gluten-Free: Yes

Dairy-Free: Yes

Vegan: Yes

2 medium fennel bulbs, sliced thin

1 can (14 oz) artichoke hearts, drained and halved or fresh artichokes, prepared

3 tablespoons olive oil

1 teaspoon fresh thyme leaves or 1/2 teaspoon dried thyme

1 teaspoon fresh rosemary, chopped or 1/2 teaspoon dried rosemary

Salt, to taste (use sea salt for AIP)

Freshly ground black pepper, to taste (omit if strictly AIP)

Heat 2 tablespoons of olive oil in a large pan over medium heat.

Put the sliced fennel in the pan and simmer for 15 to 20 minutes, turning regularly, until it softens and starts to caramelize.

To prevent shattering the artichoke hearts, add the drained artichoke hearts to the skillet and simmer for a further 10 to 15 minutes, stirring occasionally.

Season with salt, pepper, rosemary, and thyme, if using. Pour in the last tablespoon of olive oil and mix everything together.

Allow the flavors to combine by cooking for a further five minutes.

Take off the stove and serve warm as an accompaniment.

Turmeric-Roasted Cauliflower Rice

(per serving)

Serving Size: About 1 cup

Calories: 100

Fats: 7g

Carbs: 10g

Protein: 3g

Sugars: 2g

Gluten-Free: Yes

Dairy-Free: Yes

Vegan: Yes

AIP Compliant: Yes (omit black pepper)

1 medium head of cauliflower (about 4 cups riced)

1 tablespoon fresh turmeric root, grated or 1 teaspoon ground turmeric

2 tablespoons olive oil (or coconut oil)

1 teaspoon salt (or to taste)

1/2 teaspoon black pepper (omit for strict AIP)

1/4 cup fresh herbs (parsley or cilantro, chopped)

Set the oven's temperature to 425°F (220°C).

Cut the cauliflower into florets after removing the stalk and leaves. In a food processor, pulse the florets until they start to resemble rice grains. An alternative is to use a box grater to grind the cauliflower.

Grated turmeric, riced cauliflower, olive oil, salt, and black pepper (if used) should all be combined in a big dish. Toss to coat the cauliflower evenly.

Line a baking sheet with parchment paper and spread the cauliflower mixture in one layer. Roast the cauliflower in a warm oven for 20 to 25 minutes, tossing halfway through, until it is soft and beginning to turn brown.

Before serving, take the cauliflower rice out of the oven after it has roasted and top it with some fresh herbs..

Wild Mushroom and Herb

(per serving)

Serving Size: 1 cup

Calories: 120

Fats: 10g

Carbs: 8g

Protein: 3g

Sugars: 2g

Gluten-Free: Yes

Dairy-Free: Yes

Vegan: Yes

2 cups wild mushrooms (chanterelles, shiitake, or oyster mushrooms), cleaned and sliced

2 tablespoons olive oil (or coconut oil for AIP)

2 cloves garlic, minced

1 tablespoon fresh thyme, chopped

1 tablespoon fresh parsley, chopped

1 tablespoon fresh rosemary, chopped

Salt to taste (optional, use sparingly for AIP)

1 tablespoon truffle oil (for finishing)

Heat the coconut oil or olive oil in a big pan over medium heat.

Carefully avoid burning the minced garlic as you sauté it for around 30 seconds until it becomes aromatic.

Put the wild mushrooms onto the pan after cutting them into slices. Stirring periodically, sauté the mushrooms for 5 to 7 minutes, or until they are browned and soft.

Add the fresh thyme, parsley, rosemary, and salt (if using) once the mushrooms are cooked. Cook for a further two minutes after stirring to blend.

Take off the heat and cover the mushroom mélange with the truffle oil. Toss to ensure even coating.

Spoon onto a platter and savor warm.

Roasted Bone Marrow with Parsley Salad

(per serving, assuming 2 bones and salad)

Serving Size: 2 marrow bones with salad

Calories: 320

Fats: 30g

Carbs: 4g

Protein: 14g

Sugars: 0g

Gluten-Free: Yes

Dairy-Free: Yes

Vegan: No

4 beef marrow bones (cut lengthwise)

Salt and pepper (to taste, omit if following strict AIP)

1 tablespoon olive oil (optional, for drizzling)

For the Parsley Salad:

1 cup fresh parsley, finely chopped

1 tablespoon fresh lemon juice

1 tablespoon olive oil

1 clove garlic, minced (optional, omit if sensitive)

Salt (to taste, omit if following strict AIP

The first step is to preheat the oven to 450°F (232°C).

The marrow bones should be prepared by placing them on a baking sheet. Lightly season with salt and pepper (if used) and sprinkle with olive oil if preferred.

In the oven, roast the bones for about 15-20 minutes, or until the marrow is tender and starts to boil and become golden.

Make the parsley salad while the bones roast. Add the chopped parsley, lemon juice, olive oil, salt, and garlic (if using) to a bowl. Toss thoroughly to mix.

After roasting, take the bones out of the oven. Before serving, let cool a little. Using a spoon, remove the marrow and serve it with the parsley salad.

Side Dishes and Small Bites

Green Tea Kombucha-Fermented Radishes

(per serving, about 1/2 cup)

Serving Size: 1/2 cup

Calories: 15

Fats: 0g

Carbs: 3g

Protein: 0.5g

Sugars: 1g (naturally occurring)

Gluten-Free: Yes

Dairy-Free: Yes

Vegan: Yes)

1 bunch (about 8-10) fresh radishes, trimmed and sliced

1 cup green tea kombucha (store-bought or homemade)

1 teaspoon fresh ginger, grated

1 teaspoon sea salt

Rinse and trim the radishes, then cut them into thin slices. If you want consistent slices, you may use a mandoline.

Place the sea salt, grated ginger, and sliced radishes in a clean glass container. Cover the radishes with the green tea kombucha, making sure they are well covered.

Cover the jar with cheesecloth fastened with a rubber band or seal it with a lid. Depending on your taste, let it ferment for three to five days at room temperature (preferably between 70°F and 75°F).

Examine the radishes' taste and tanginess three days later. For a more intense taste, keep fermenting for up to five days.

Put the radishes in the fridge after they have fermented to your desired consistency. They keep their taste in the refrigerator and may be eaten cold.

Turmeric-Ginger Sauerkraut

(per serving, based on 1 tablespoon serving size)

Serving Size: 1 tablespoon

Calories: 8

Fats: 0g

Carbs: 2g

Protein: 0g

Sugars: 0g

Gluten-Free: Yes

Dairy-Free: Yes

Vegan: Yes

AIP Compliant: Yes (if black peppercorns are omitted)

1 medium head of purple cabbage (about 2 pounds)

1 tablespoon fresh turmeric root, grated

1 tablespoon fresh ginger root, grated

1 tablespoon sea salt (preferably non-iodized)

1 teaspoon whole black peppercorns (optional, omit for strict AIP)

Filtered water (if needed, to cover)

Take off any outer leaves that are damaged. Slice the cabbage thinly after cutting it in quarters and removing the core (or shred it with a food processor or mandoline).

Add the sea salt, grated ginger, grated turmeric, and sliced cabbage to a large bowl. For five to ten minutes, rub the cabbage with salt using your hands until its juices begin to flow. This aids in the production of the brine required for fermentation.

Pour the cabbage mixture into a glass jar (about a quart size) that has been cleaned and disinfected. Make sure the cabbage is completely covered by its own liquid by packing it down firmly. Give the jar's top an inch or so of headroom.

If the cabbage isn't completely immersed, cover it with a little filtered water.

Cover the jar with a cover that is just loose enough to let the gasses out. For one to two weeks, let the jar ferment in a cool, dark location (preferably between 65 and 75°F or 18 and 24°C). Make sure the cabbage stays immersed every day, and after a week, taste it to determine the proper level of tanginess.

Tighten the cover and put the jar in the fridge after it has matured to your preference. You may eat the sauerkraut right away, but it becomes better after a few days in the refrigerator.

Coconut Water Kefir with Lavender

(per serving)

Serving Size: 1 cup (approximately 8 oz)

Calories: 45

Fats: 0g

Carbs: 9g

Protein: 1g

Sugars: 6g

Gluten-Free: Yes

Dairy-Free: Yes

Vegan: Yes

4 cups coconut water (preferably fresh and natural)

1 tablespoon kefir grains

1 tablespoon dried lavender flowers

The first step is to prepare the coconut water by pouring it into a clean glass jar, allowing room at the top for fermentation.

Mix the coconut water with the kefir grains.

Stir the dried lavender flowers gently.

Use a fresh towel or a coffee filter fastened with a rubber band to cover the jar. Depending on your taste, leave it at room temperature (around 68–85°F or 20–29°C) for 24–48 hours. It will become tangier the longer it ferments.

Use cheesecloth or a fine mesh strainer to remove the lavender flowers and kefir grains once the mixture has fermented to your preference. The kefir grains may be stored for use in later batches.

Pour the kefir into a jar or a clean glass container and put it in the refrigerator. It may be kept for up to a week or eaten right away.

Fermented Green Papaya Relish

(per serving, about 1/4 cup)

Serving Size: 1/4 cup

Calories: 20

Fats: 0g

Carbs: 5g

Protein: 0.5g

Sugars: 1g

Gluten-Free: Yes

Dairy-Free: Yes

Vegan: Yes

2 cups shredded green papaya

1 teaspoon sea salt

1 tablespoon fresh ginger, grated

1/4 cup fresh cilantro, chopped

Peel and shred the green papaya first. To get fine shreds, you may use a food processor or a box grater.

Add the chopped cilantro, grated ginger, sea salt, and shredded green papaya to a large mixing dish. To guarantee that the salt is dispersed evenly, carefully mix.

Pour the mixture into a sanitized glass container that is airtight. To eliminate air pockets, pack it firmly, leaving an inch or so at the top.

Depending on the desired level of sourness, keep the jar at room temperature for 3–7 days after loosely sealing it to enable gasses to escape. To maintain the mixture immersed in its own liquid, check it every day and apply pressure.

Taste the relish after the fermenting time. Once the desired level of sourness has been achieved, securely shut the jar and place it in the refrigerator. You may keep it in the refrigerator for up to two weeks.

.

Pickled Watermelon Radish

(per serving, about 1/4 cup)

Serving Size: 1/4 cup

Calories: 25

Fats: 0g

Carbs: 6g

Protein: 1g

Sugars: 1g

Gluten-Free: Yes

Dairy-Free: Yes

Vegan: Yes

2 medium watermelon radishes, thinly sliced

1 cup apple cider vinegar (raw, unfiltered)

1 cup water

1 tablespoon sea salt

2 bay leaves

1 teaspoon pink peppercorns

1 tablespoon honey (optional, adjust to taste)

Put the water, sea salt, apple cider vinegar, and honey (if using) in a saucepan. Heat until the salt dissolves, over medium heat. Take off the heat and let it reach room temperature.

Use a mandoline or a sharp knife to finely slice the watermelon radishes while the brine cools.

Arrange the pink peppercorns, bay leaves, and sliced watermelon radishes in a sanitized glass jar.

Pour the chilled brine over the radishes in the container, making sure they are well immersed. To keep them immersed, you may need to use a clean piece of parchment paper or a little weight.

Tightly seal the jar and let it ferment for two to three days at room temperature. After two days, taste the radishes, and if you want a stronger flavor, let them ferment longer.

Refrigerate the pickled watermelon radish after the fermentation is complete. They will gain more taste with time, but they may be eaten right now.

Beet Kvass with Citrus

(per serving, assuming 8 servings from the recipe)

Serving Size: 1 cup

Calories: 15

Fats: 0g

Carbs: 4g

Protein: 0g

Sugars: 1g

Gluten-Free:Yes

Dairy-Free: Yes (if whey is omitted)

Vegan: Yes (if whey is omitted)

2 medium beets, peeled and chopped

4 cups filtered water

1 tablespoon sea salt

Peel of 1 organic orange (avoid the white pith)

1 star anise pod

1 tablespoon whey (optional, for fermentation; omit for strict AIP)

Put the diced beets in a large fermenting container or glass jar.

Fill the jar with the filtered water, sea salt, orange peel, star anise, and whey (if using).

To dissolve the salt, thoroughly stir the mixture.

To let air out while keeping impurities out, cover the jar with a clean cloth or a fermentation lid. For three to five days, keep the jar at room temperature. Taste every day; a tart flavor should emerge.

Strain off the star anise, orange peel, and beets once it has fermented to your preferred consistency. Store the kvass in the refrigerator after pouring it into a jar or clean glass container.

Probiotic-Rich Carrot Sticks

(per serving, about 1/2 cup)

Serving Size: 1/2 cup (about 4-5 sticks)

Calories: 30

Fats: 0g

Carbs: 7g

Protein: 1g

Sugars: 3g

Gluten-Free: Yes

Dairy-Free: Yes

Vegan: Yes

1 lb rainbow carrots or regular carrots

3-4 cloves garlic, crushed

1 teaspoon fresh thyme leaves

1 tablespoon sea salt

Filtered water (to cover the carrots)

The rainbow carrots should be peeled and sliced into sticks or rounds that are around 3–4 inches long.

Tightly pack the carrot sticks in a sanitized glass jar, allowing a gap of about 1 inch at the top.

Fill the jar with the carrots and add the smashed garlic cloves and fresh thyme.

The brine is made by dissolving sea salt in purified water. Cover the carrots with the brine until they are completely immersed. Give the jar's top an inch or so of room.

Place a cover on the jar or a fresh cloth fastened with a rubber band. For five to seven days, let it sit at room temperature, preferably at 70°F or 21°C. Press down to keep the carrots buried and check every day.

Taste the carrots five to seven days later. If the tanginess is to your liking, put them in the fridge to delay the fermentation process. Give them a few more days to ferment if you want a stronger taste.

Charred Sunchokes with Sage

(per serving)

Serving Size: About 1 cup

Calories: 160

Fats: 8g

Carbs: 20g

Protein: 3g

Sugars: 1g

Gluten-Free: Yes

Dairy-Free: Yes

Vegan: Yes

AIP-Friendly: Yes (omit pepper)

1 pound Jerusalem artichokes (sunchokes), scrubbed and sliced

2 tablespoons olive oil

1 teaspoon fresh sage, chopped or 1/2 teaspoon dried sage

Salt and pepper to taste (omit for strict AIP)

1 tablespoon lemon juice (optional, for added flavor)

Set the oven's temperature to 425°F (220°C).

Place the sliced Jerusalem artichokes in a mixing basin and toss with chopped sage, olive oil, salt, and pepper (if using).

Line a baking sheet with parchment paper and arrange the sunchokes in a single layer. Bake for 25 to 30 minutes, turning them halfway through, or until they are charred on the edges and golden brown.

Take out of the oven and, if you'd like, pour some lemon juice over it. Gently toss to mix.

Spoon onto a platter and serve hot..

Grilled Japanese Sweet Potatoes with Rosemary

(per serving, based on 4 servings)

Serving Size: 1 medium sweet potato

Calories: 180

Fats: 6g

Carbs: 35g

Protein: 3g

Sugars: 7g

Gluten-Free: Yes

Dairy-Free: Yes

Vegan: Yes

4 medium purple-skinned Japanese sweet potatoes

2 tablespoons olive oil (or avocado oil)

2 cloves garlic, minced

2 tablespoons fresh rosemary, chopped

Salt (to taste, optional)

The first step is to preheat your grill to medium-high heat, which is around 375°F to 400°F (190°C to 204°C).

Thoroughly wash and clean the sweet potatoes. They have additional nutrients when the skin is left on, but you may peel them if you'd like.

To ensure consistent cooking, cut the sweet potatoes into rounds or wedges that are 1/2 inch thick.

Add the olive oil, chopped rosemary, minced garlic, and salt (if needed) to a large bowl. Toss in the sweet potatoes until they are well covered in the mixture.

Arrange the sweet potato slices in a single layer on the grill. They should be tender and have lovely grill marks after grilling for 5 to 7 minutes on each side. Depending on how thick the slices are, you may need to change the cooking time.

Take off the grill and serve warm, topped with more rosemary if you want.

Roasted Celeriac with Thyme

(per serving, serves 4)

Serving Size: 1/4 of the recipe

Calories: 90

Fats: 6g

Carbohydrates: 10g

Protein: 1g

Sugars: 2g

Gluten-Free: Yes

Dairy-Free: Yes

Vegan: Yes

1 medium celeriac root, peeled and cubed (about 2 cups)

2 tablespoons olive oil

1 teaspoon herbes de Provence

Salt, to taste (optional)

Fresh thyme leaves, for garnish (optional)

Set the oven temperature to 400°F (200°C).

Put the cubed celeriac, olive oil, herbs de Provence, and salt (if using) in a mixing bowl. Toss well to evenly coat every item.

Arrange the celeriac cubes in a single layer on a parchment paper-lined baking sheet. To ensure equal cooking, stir halfway through and roast for 30 to 35 minutes, or until golden brown and soft.

When ready to serve, take it out of the oven, add some fresh thyme leaves if you want, and serve it warm.

.

Grilled Radicchio with Oregano

(per serving)

Serving Size: 1 quartered head of radicchio

Calories: 90

Fats: 8g

Carbs: 6g

Protein: 2g

Sugars: 1g

Gluten-Free: Yes

Dairy-Free: Yes

Vegan: Yes

2 heads of radicchio (quartered)

2 tablespoons olive oil

2 tablespoons fresh oregano, chopped or 1 tablespoon dried oregano

Salt and pepper (to taste, optional)

Set the grill's temperature to medium-high.

Place the quartered radicchio in a big bowl, drizzle with olive oil, and top with chopped oregano. Toss to ensure even coating. Add salt and pepper if you'd like (but only if it's within your dietary restrictions).

Lay the quarters of the radicchio on the grill, cut-side down. They should be soft and faintly browned after grilling for 4–5 minutes on each side.

Take off the grill and serve warm, topped with more oregano if you want and drizzled with any leftover olive oil.

Roasted Kabocha Squash with Lavender

(per serving, serves 4)

Serving Size: 1/4 of the recipe

Calories: 150

Fats: 6g

Carbs: 22g

Protein: 2g

Sugars: 6g (from maple syrup and natural sugars in squash)

Gluten-Free: Yes

Dairy-Free: Yes

Vegan: Yes

1 medium kabocha squash

1 tablespoon dried culinary lavender

2 tablespoons maple syrup

2 tablespoons olive oil

Salt (to taste; optional)

The first step is to preheat the oven to 400°F (200°C).

Split the squash in two and remove the seeds.

Cut the squash into cubes or wedges that are about 1 inch thick.

Combine the dried lavender and olive oil in a small basin. To infuse the lavender taste into the oil, let it rest for around ten minutes.

Toss the squash wedges in the olive oil scented with lavender in a large mixing basin until they are well covered.

To guarantee uniform coating, drizzle the squash with maple syrup and toss once more.

Sprinkle with a touch of salt if you'd like.

To roast the squash, arrange the squash wedges in a single layer on a parchment paper-lined baking sheet.

Squash should be soft and caramelized after 25 to 30 minutes of roasting in a preheated oven; turn halfway through to ensure equal cooking.

Before serving, take it out of the oven and allow it to cool somewhat. Savor it warm as an accompaniment

Grilled Baby Bok Choy with Ginger

(per serving)

Serving Size: 2 halves (1 bok choy)

Calories: 30

Fats: 1g

Carbs: 6g

Protein: 1g

Sugars: 1g

Gluten-Free: Yes

Dairy-Free: Yes

Vegan: Yes

4 baby bok choy, halved lengthwise

2 tablespoons coconut aminos

1 tablespoon fresh ginger, grated

1 tablespoon olive oil (optional, for grilling)

Salt (to taste, optional)

Set your grill or grill pan to medium heat.

Combine the grated ginger and coconut aminos in a small dish.

Season with salt and, if needed, brush the bok choy halves with olive oil. Make sure the bok choy is well covered by drizzling it with the coconut aminos and ginger combination.

Lay the halves of bok choy cut side down on the grill. The leaves should be slightly wilted and the edges should be browned after 3–4 minutes on the grill.

After flipping the bok choy, grill it for a further two to three minutes, or until it is crisp but still soft.

Take off the grill, then serve warm as an accompaniment..

Kohlrabi Carpaccio

(per serving, serves 2)

Serving Size: 1/2 recipe

Calories: 120

Fats: 10g

Carbs: 8g

Protein: 2g

Sugars: 3g

Gluten-Free: Yes

Dairy-Free: Yes

Vegan: Yes

1 large kohlrabi, peeled and thinly sliced

2 tablespoons olive oil

2 tablespoons fresh herbs (parsley, basil, or dill), finely chopped

Juice of 1 lemon

Salt and pepper to taste (omit pepper if following strict AIP)

Red pepper flakes for a bit of heat

Using a sharp knife or mandoline, carefully slice the kohlrabi into uniform, thin rounds after peeling it.

Whisk together the lemon juice, olive oil, chopped herbs, and a bit of salt (and pepper, if needed) in a small dish.

To create a beautiful presentation, place the kohlrabi slices on a serving dish, gently overlapping them.

Coat the kohlrabi slices equally with the dressing by drizzling it over them.

To let the flavors combine, let it rest for 5 to 10 minutes. You may serve it cold or warm.

.

Jicama and Green Apple Slaw

(per serving)

Serving Size: Approximately 1 cup

Calories: 60

Fats: 0.5g

Carbs: 15g

Protein: 1g

Sugars: 6g

Gluten-Free: Yes

Dairy-Free: Yes

Vegan: Yes

1 medium jicama, peeled and julienned

1 large green apple, cored and julienned (such as Granny Smith)

1/4 cup fresh mint leaves, finely chopped

Juice of 2 limes

Salt to taste (optional)

First, get the vegetables ready by peeling and julienneing the jicama. Core the green apple and julienne it.

Put the green apple and julienned jicama in a big bowl.

Add the freshly cut mint leaves.

In order to dress the slaw, squeeze the lime juice over the mixture and stir everything well. If desired, add salt for seasoning.

Before serving, let the slaw chill in the fridge for 10 to 15 minutes for the greatest taste.

Savor as a light snack or as a cool side dish.

Roasted Bone Marrow with Parsley

(per serving, based on 2 bone halves)

Serving Size: 2 bone halves

Calories: 300

Fats: 28g

Carbs: 2g

Protein: 15g

Sugars: 0g

Gluten-Free: Yes

Dairy-Free: Yes

Vegan: No

4-6 grass-fed beef marrow bones (cut lengthwise)

Sea salt (to taste)

1 cup fresh parsley, finely chopped

1 tablespoon olive oil (optional, for drizzling)

Lemon wedges (for serving, optional)

The first step is to preheat the oven to 450°F (232°C).

Arrange the marrow bones in an upright position on a parchment paper-lined baking sheet. Season the bones with a little sea salt if you want

For about 15-20 minutes, or until the marrow is tender and starts to separate from the bone, roast the bones in a preheated oven. It should be gently browned on top.

In a bowl, mix the chopped parsley, a sprinkling of sea salt, and a drizzle of olive oil (if needed) while the bones roast. Toss to mix.

Take the bones out of the oven and let them cool a little. If preferred, serve the roasted marrow with lemon wedges to squeeze over it and the parsley salad on the side.

Rutabaga "Rice" Pilaf

(per serving)

Serving Size: 1 cup

Calories: 130

Fats: 8g

Carbs: 14g

Protein: 2g

Sugars: 3g

Gluten-Free: Yes

Dairy-Free: Yes

Vegan: Yes

2 cups rutabaga, riced (about 1 medium rutabaga)

2 tablespoons olive oil

1 small onion, finely chopped

2 cloves garlic, minced

1 teaspoon fresh thyme, chopped or ½ teaspoon dried thyme

1 teaspoon fresh rosemary, chopped or ½ teaspoon dried rosemary

1/2 teaspoon sea salt (adjust to taste)

1/4 teaspoon black pepper (optional, omit for strict AIP)

1/4 cup parsley, chopped (for garnish)

Cut the rutabaga into pieces after peeling it. Rice the rutabaga in a food processor or box grater until it looks like rice.

Heat the olive oil in a big skillet over a medium heat. Sauté the chopped onion and garlic for three to four minutes, or until the onion is aromatic and transparent.

To cook the rutabaga, add it to the pan with the rice and toss to mix. Add salt, pepper (if using), rosemary, and thyme for seasoning. Cook, stirring occasionally, until the rutabaga is soft but still slightly hard, approximately 10 to 12 minutes.

Take off the heat and add the chopped parsley as a garnish before serving. Serve warm as a basis for your main entrée or as a side dish.

Purslane and Watercress Salad

(per serving)

Serving Size: 1 salad (makes about 4 servings)

Calories: 80

Fats: 7g

Carbs: 6g

Protein: 2g

Sugars: 1g

Gluten-Free: Yes

Dairy-Free: Yes

Vegan: Yes

2 cups fresh purslane, rinsed and chopped

2 cups fresh watercress, rinsed and trimmed

2 tablespoons extra virgin olive oil

Juice of 1 lemon

Salt and pepper to taste (optional)

Put the chopped watercress and purslane in a big basin.

Whisk the lemon juice and olive oil in a small dish. If using, add salt and pepper.

Drizzle the greens with the dressing and gently mix to mix.

Spoon salad into dishes and eat right away

Braised Artichoke Hearts

(per serving)

Serving Size: 1 cup

Calories: 150

Fats: 8g

Carbs: 15g

Protein: 5g

Sugars: 1g

4 fresh artichoke hearts (trimmed and quartered)

2 cups bone broth (preferably homemade or low-sodium)

2 tablespoons olive oil

2 cloves garlic, minced (optional)

1 teaspoon fresh thyme or 1/2 teaspoon dried thyme

1 teaspoon fresh rosemary or 1/2 teaspoon dried rosemary

Salt to taste (use sea salt if desired)

Gluten-Free: Yes

Dairy-Free: Yes

Vegan: No (due to bone broth)

Cut the artichoke hearts into quarters after trimming them off the rough ends and outer leaves.

Heat the olive oil in a big saucepan or skillet over medium heat. If using, add the minced garlic and cook for one to two minutes, or until fragrant.

Toss in the quartered artichoke hearts and cook for a further three to four minutes, stirring now and again.

Incorporate the bone broth, salt, thyme, and rosemary. Heat the mixture until it simmers gently.

Lower the heat to low and cover the pan. For 20 to 25 minutes, or until the artichokes are soft and have absorbed some of the broth's aromas, let them braise.

Take off the heat and serve warm as a light main course or as a side dish.

Sea Vegetable Salad

(per serving)

Serving Size: 1 salad

Calories: 90

Fats: 7g

Carbs: 8g

Protein: 2g

Sugars: 1g

Gluten-Free: Yes

Dairy-Free: Yes

Vegan: Yes

1 cup mixed seaweeds (dulse, wakame, and sea lettuce, rehydrated if dried)

1 tablespoon sesame oil

1 teaspoon fresh ginger, grated

1 tablespoon lime juice

Salt to taste (optional)

1/4 cup sliced cucumber

If you're using dried seaweeds, rehydrate them as directed on the box (typically by soaking them in water for 10 to 15 minutes). After draining, cut into small pieces.

Combine the lime juice, sesame oil, grated ginger, and salt (if using) in a small dish.

Put the sliced cucumber (if using) and rehydrated seaweeds in a big bowl. Drizzle the salad with the dressing and carefully mix to evenly coat the seaweeds.

Snacks and Smoothies

Cassava Flour Breakfast Bars

(per bar, makes approximately 12 bars)

Serving Size: 1 bar

Calories: 130

Fats: 5g

Carbs: 22g

Protein: 2g

Sugars: 7g

Gluten-Free: Yes

Dairy-Free: Yes

Nut-Free: Yes

Vegan: Yes

1 cup cassava flour

1/2 cup tigernut flour

1/2 cup shredded coconut (unsweetened)

1 cup dried figs, chopped

1/4 cup maple syrup

1 teaspoon ground cinnamon

1/4 teaspoon salt

1/4 cup water (as needed)

Line an 8 × 8-inch baking dish with parchment paper and preheat your oven to 350°F (175°C).

Put the cassava flour, tigernut flour, chopped dried figs, crushed cinnamon, salt, and shredded coconut in a large mixing bowl.

Mix the dry ingredients well with the maple syrup. A spoonful of water at a time should be added gradually until the mixture stays together without becoming too moist.

Fill the baking dish with the mixture and level the bottom of the dish.

Bake for 25 to 30 minutes, or until the center is set and the sides are golden brown.

After letting the bars cool in the pan for around ten minutes, use the parchment paper to remove them. Before cutting them into squares, allow them to cool fully on a wire rack.

Sweet Potato "Toast" Squares

(per serving; 2 slices)

Serving Size: 2 slices

Calories: 220

Fats: 14g

Carbs: 36g

Protein: 2g

Sugars: 6g

2 medium sweet potatoes

1/4 cup coconut butter (softened)

1 teaspoon ground cinnamon

Pinch of sea salt (optional)

Gluten-Free: Yes

Dairy-Free: Yes

Vegan: Yes

Set the oven temperature to 400°F (200°C).

Give them a good wash and scrub. Cut them into 1/4-inch thick lengthwise slices.

To bake sweet potatoes, arrange the slices on a parchment paper-lined baking sheet. Bake, turning halfway through, for 25 to 30 minutes, or until soft and beginning to caramelize.

As the sweet potatoes bake, prepare the topping by combining the coconut butter, ground cinnamon, and sea salt (if using) in a small dish.

After baking, take the sweet potato slices out of the oven and let them cool a little. Cover each slice with the cinnamon-coconut butter mixture.

Savor them right away or allow them to cool fully for a snack that can be carried about.

Turmeric Chicken Collard Wraps

(per serving, 2 wraps)

Serving Size: 2 wraps

Calories: 380

Fats: 22g

Carbs: 18g

Protein: 32g

Sugars: 2g

Gluten-Free: Yes

Dairy-Free: Yes

Paleo: Yes

AIP: Yes

1 pound boneless, skinless chicken breast

1 tablespoon turmeric powder

1 teaspoon garlic powder

1 teaspoon onion powder

1 tablespoon olive oil (or coconut oil)

1/2 teaspoon sea salt

1/2 teaspoon black pepper (omit if strictly AIP)

4 large collard green leaves

1 ripe avocado, sliced

1 tablespoon fresh ginger, grated

Juice of 1 lime

Fresh herbs for garnish (optional, cilantro or parsley)

Put the turmeric, sea salt, onion powder, garlic powder, and black pepper (if using) in a bowl.

Evenly rub the chicken breasts with the spice mixture.

In a skillet over medium heat, heat the olive oil. Add chicken breasts that have been seasoned.

Cook until the chicken is cooked through and the internal temperature reaches 165°F (75°C), approximately 6-7 minutes each side. Before slicing, take off the heat and let it cool for a few minutes.

Bring a big saucepan of water to a boil while the chicken cools. To halt the cooking process, place the collard leaves in an ice bath after

blanching them for approximately 30 seconds to soften them. Use paper towels to pat dry.

Place a piece of sliced chicken in the middle of a collard leaf that has been laid flat. Add slices of avocado, grated ginger, and lime juice on top.

Tightly roll the collard leaf from bottom to top after folding the edges over the filling.

Continue with the remaining filling and collard leaves. If preferred, top with fresh herbs and serve right away.

Roasted Carrot and Ginger Energy Balls

(per serving)

Serving Size: 1 energy ball (makes about 12 balls)

Calories: 80

Fats: 2g

Carbs: 18g

Protein: 1g

Sugars: 10g (naturally occurring from dates and carrots)

Gluten-Free: Yes

Dairy-Free: Yes

Nut-Free: Yes

Vegan: Yes (if collagen peptides are plant-based)

1 cup roasted carrots (approximately 2 medium carrots)

1 cup Medjool dates, pitted

1 tablespoon fresh ginger, grated

1/2 cup unsweetened shredded coconut

1/4 cup collagen peptides

1/2 teaspoon cinnamon (optional)

First, roast the carrots. Set the oven's temperature to 400°F, or 200°C. Cut the carrots into little pieces after peeling them. Roast for 25 to 30 minutes, or until soft, after tossing with a little amount of olive oil (optional). Let it cool.

Grated ginger, shredded coconut, Medjool dates, roasted carrots, collagen peptides, and cinnamon (if used) should all be combined in a food processor. Pulse until the mixture begins to cling to one another and is well mixed. It may be necessary to repeatedly scrape down the bowl's sides.

Using your hands, roll the mixture into tiny balls that are approximately one inch in diameter once it has been well mixed.

To firm up, place the energy balls on a baking sheet coated with parchment and place them in the refrigerator for at least half an hour.

Savor it right now or keep it in the fridge for up to a week in an airtight jar.

Salmon Patties with Herbs

(per serving, 2 patties)

Serving Size: 2 patties

Calories: 330

Fats: 17g

Carbs: 26g

Protein: 24g

Sugars: 3g

Gluten-Free: Yes

Dairy-Free: Yes

Egg-Free: Yes

Nut-Free: Yes

Paleo: Yes

1 pound wild-caught salmon, skinless and boneless

1 medium sweet potato, cooked and mashed (about 1 cup)

1/4 cup fresh herbs (parsley, dill, or chives), finely chopped

1 tablespoon gelatin powder

1 teaspoon garlic powder

1/2 teaspoon onion powder

Salt (to taste, optional)

Pepper (to taste, optional)

Coconut oil or olive oil

Boil or bake the sweet potato until it is tender. Peel and mash it till it's smooth after cooking.

Use a fork to flake the salmon in a big bowl. Add the gelatin, fresh herbs, mashed sweet potato, onion and garlic powders, and salt and pepper (if using). Stir until well blended.

The next step is to form patties. To do this, divide the ingredients into equal pieces and form each into around eight patties.

You may chill the patties for half an hour before cooking them to improve binding.

Heat olive or coconut oil in a pan over medium heat. Add the patties and fry until golden brown and well cooked, approximately 4–5 minutes each side.

After taking the patties out of the pan, place them on paper towels to drain. Warm or room temperature, serve.

Maca Root Recovery Smoothie

(per serving)

Serving Size: 1 smoothie

Calories: 290

Fats: 16g

Carbs: 36g

Protein: 5g

Sugars: 12g (naturally occurring from banana)

Gluten-Free: Yes

Dairy-Free: Yes

Vegan: Yes (if collagen is omitted)

1 cup frozen cauliflower florets

1 cup coconut milk (canned or carton, unsweetened)

1 tablespoon maca powder

1 ripe banana (fresh or frozen)

1 scoop collagen powder (optional)

Put the frozen cauliflower, banana, coconut milk, maca powder, and collagen powder (if using) in a blender.

Blend on high speed until the cauliflower is completely integrated and the mixture is creamy and smooth.

If you want to add extra banana for sweetness, taste the smoothie.

Transfer the smoothie to a glass and start drinking right away.

Ashwagandha Berry Blast

(per serving)

Serving Size: 1 smoothie

Calories: 210

Fats: 9g

Carbs: 34g

Protein: 3g

Sugars: 18g (naturally occurring from berries and honey)

Gluten-Free: Yes

Dairy-Free: Yes

Vegan: Yes (if honey is omitted

1 cup mixed berries (blueberries, strawberries, raspberries, or blackberries)

1 cup coconut milk (canned or carton, unsweetened)

1 teaspoon ashwagandha powder

1 tablespoon honey (optional, adjust to taste)

1 cup fresh spinach (packed)

Wash the berries well if you are using fresh ones. Thawing is not necessary if using frozen berries.

Put the raw spinach, ashwagandha powder, coconut milk, honey (if using), and mixed berries in a blender.

Process the ingredients on high speed until it becomes creamy and smooth.

If you want the smoothie to be sweeter, taste it and add more honey.

Transfer the smoothie to a glass and start drinking right away.

Reishi Mushroom Green Smoothie

(per serving)

Serving Size: 1 smoothie

Calories: 70

Fats: 0.5g

Carbs: 16g

Protein: 1g

Sugars: 9g (naturally occurring from apple and coconut water)

Gluten-Free: Yes

Dairy-Free: Yes

Vegan: Yes

1 teaspoon reishi mushroom powder

1/2 cucumber (peeled and chopped)

1/2 green apple (cored and chopped)

1/4 cup fresh mint leaves

1 cup coconut water

To mix, put the reishi mushroom powder, cucumber, green apple, mint, and coconut water in a blender.

Blend on high until the mixture is smooth and the ingredients are fully incorporated.

Transfer the smoothie to a glass and start drinking right away.

Golden Milk Smoothie

(per serving)

Serving Size: 1 smoothie

Calories: 210

Fats: 14g

Carbs: 22g

Protein: 2g

Sugars: 12g (naturally occurring from banana)

Gluten-Free: Yes

Dairy-Free: Yes

Vegan: Yes

1 frozen banana

1/2 teaspoon ground turmeric

1/2 teaspoon fresh ginger, grated

Pinch of black pepper

1 cup coconut milk (unsweetened, from a can or carton)

1/4 teaspoon ground cardamom

Put the frozen banana, cardamom, coconut milk, black pepper, turmeric, and shredded ginger in a blender.

Process the ingredients on high speed until it becomes creamy and smooth.

Transfer the smoothie to a glass and start drinking right away.

Cordyceps Boost Smoothie

(per serving)

Serving Size: 1 smoothie

Calories: 130

Fats: 6g

Carbs: 18g

Protein: 2g

Sugars: 7g (naturally occurring from beets and maple syrup)

Gluten-Free: Yes

Dairy-Free: Yes

Vegan: Yes

1/2 teaspoon cordyceps powder

1/2 cup cooked or raw beets, chopped (cooked is milder and blends smoother)

1/2 cup carrot, chopped

1 cup coconut milk (unsweetened, from a can or carton)

1 teaspoon maple syrup (optional, adjust for sweetness)

You may choose to roast or simmer the raw beets for a little time to soften them. Although optional, this may facilitate mixing.

Put the carrots, beets, coconut milk, maple syrup, and cordyceps powder in a blender.

Process the ingredients on high speed until it becomes creamy and smooth.

Transfer the smoothie to a glass and start drinking right away.

Trail Mix

(Per 1/4 cup serving)

Calories: 180

Fats: 14g

Carbs: 12g

Protein: 4g

Sugars: 6g (naturally occurring from dried fruits)

1/2 cup Brazil nuts

1/2 cup walnuts

1/4 cup goji berries

1/4 cup mulberries

(AIP Option)

1/2 cup tigernuts

1/4 cup dried figs, chopped

1/4 cup coconut chips

Gluten-Free: Yes

Dairy-Free: Yes

Vegan: Yes

In a bowl, combine all ingredients. When creating the AIP alternative, mix together coconut chips, dried figs, and tigernuts.

Store for up to two weeks at room temperature after transferring to an airtight container.

Spiced Seed Crackers

(per serving, approximately 10 crackers)

Seed Crackers (Non-AIP):

Calories: 80

Fats: 5g

Carbs: 6g

Protein: 3g

Sugars: 0g (naturally occurring)

Cassava Crackers (AIP Alternative):

Calories: 90

Fats: 4g

Carbs: 12g

Protein: 1g

Sugars: 0g

Gluten-Free: Yes

Dairy-Free: Yes

Vegan: Yes

Seed Cracker Version (Non-AIP):

1/2 cup flax seeds

1/4 cup chia seeds

1 teaspoon dried herbs (e.g. rosemary, thyme, or oregano)

1/2 teaspoon garlic powder

1/4 teaspoon sea salt

1/2 cup water

AIP Alternative (Cassava Flour Crackers):

1/2 cup cassava flour

1 tablespoon olive oil

1 teaspoon dried herbs (same as above)

1/2 teaspoon garlic powder

1/4 teaspoon sea salt

1/4 cup water

For Non-AIP Seed Crackers:

Set the oven's temperature to 300°F (150°C). Put parchment paper on a baking pan.

Put the herbs, garlic powder, water, chia seeds, flax seeds, and salt in a mixing dish. To give the mixture time to thicken, let it rest for ten minutes.

Evenly distribute the ingredients to a thickness of about 1/8 inch on the parchment paper. Bake, turning halfway through, until crisp, 30 to 35 minutes.

Allow to cool before slicing.

AIP-Compliant: Cassava cracker version only	**Regarding Cassava Crackers (AIP Substitute):** **Set the oven's temperature to 325°F (165°C). Put parchment paper on a baking pan.** **Put the herbs, garlic powder, olive oil, salt, and cassava flour in a mixing bowl. Add water gradually while mixing to produce a dough.** **Roll, then bake: Between two parchment papers sheets, roll out the dough to a thickness of about 1/8 inch. Transfer to the baking sheet, cut into squares, and bake for 20 to 25 minutes, or until crisp and golden.** **Before serving, let it cool fully.**

Maple Cinnamon Granola

(per 1/4-cup serving)

Calories: 150

Fats: 12g

Carbs: 10g

Protein: 2g

Sugars: 5g (from natural maple syrup)

Gluten-Free: Yes

Dairy-Free: Yes

Vegan: Yes

For Anti-Inflammatory Diet:

1 cup pecans, chopped

1/2 cup pumpkin seeds

1/2 cup unsweetened coconut flakes

1 teaspoon ground cinnamon

2 tablespoons maple syrup

For AIP Diet Alternative:

1 cup unsweetened coconut flakes

1 cup tigernuts, chopped

1/2 cup dried apple chunks (unsweetened)

1 teaspoon ground cinnamon

2 tablespoons maple syrup

Set the oven's temperature to 325°F (165°C). Put parchment paper on a baking pan.

For the anti-inflammatory version, mix the pecans, pumpkin seeds, coconut flakes, and cinnamon in a big bowl (or, for the AIP version, add the coconut flakes, tigernuts, dried apple pieces, and cinnamon).

Pour the maple syrup on top of the mixture and whisk until everything is covered.

Line the prepared baking sheet with a uniform layer of the granola mixture. Bake until brown and aromatic, stirring halfway through to avoid burning, 15 to 20 minutes.

Before serving, let the granola cool fully on the baking pan. As it cools, the granola will get crispier.

Keep for up to a week in an airtight container

Golden Turmeric Nut Mix

(per 1/4 cup serving)

Calories: 180

Fats: 16g

Carbs: 6g

Protein: 4g

Sugars: 1g (naturally occurring)

Gluten-Free: Yes

Dairy-Free: Yes

Vegan: Yes

1 cup raw almonds

1 cup raw walnuts

1/2 cup unsweetened coconut flakes

1 teaspoon ground turmeric

1/4 teaspoon freshly ground black pepper

1/2 teaspoon sea salt

1 tablespoon coconut oil (melted)

Set the oven's temperature to 325°F (165°C).

Put the almonds, walnuts, and coconut flakes in a big basin.

Combine the sea salt, black pepper, and turmeric in a small bowl. Cover the nut mixture with the melted coconut oil, and then top with the spice mixture. To guarantee that every component is covered equally, toss well.

Line a baking sheet with parchment paper and evenly distribute the nut mix. Bake until the nuts are aromatic and brown, stirring halfway through, 12 to 15 minutes.

Before serving, let the mixture cool fully. Keep for up to a week at room temperature in an airtight container.

Turmeric Plantain Chips as an Alternative to AIP

1 cup roasted plantain chips - For a crispy, filling snack, toss with 1/2 teaspoon turmeric and a pinch of sea salt.

For those following the AIP diet, keep in mind that all nuts and seeds should be avoided during the elimination period. The offered AIP substitutes adhere to the rules of the protocol. You may try the dishes based on nuts and seeds as you reintroduce meals.

PART 5: Lifestyle Tips for Managing Inflammatory Flare Ups

Stress's Impact on Autoimmune Health

Your body produces stress hormones like cortisol and adrenaline when you're under stress. When stress becomes chronic, these hormones may cause chronic inflammation, although they are helpful in short-term situations (such as when you need to respond fast to danger). This ongoing stress may exacerbate symptoms for those with autoimmune diseases, making it more difficult to manage flare-ups. The equilibrium of your gut microbiome, a community of bacteria essential to digestion and immune system function, may be upset by prolonged stress.

According to research, "leaky gut" syndrome—a disease in which the gut lining becomes more porous, enabling potentially dangerous chemicals to enter the bloodstream—can result from an imbalance in the gut microbiota, which is often brought on by stress. Your immune system may overreact as a result, resulting in inflammation. Therefore, stress management may promote gut health and lower inflammation in addition to making you feel peaceful.

Autoimmune Health Stress Management Strategies

Using stress-reduction strategies that suit your requirements is crucial to successfully lowering inflammation. The following useful, approachable techniques are simple to adopt into everyday life:

1. Deep breathing lowers the release of stress hormones by telling your body that it's okay to relax. This easy exercise may boost immunity, ease stress, and decrease blood pressure.
    - Try "box breathing," which involves taking a deep breath for four counts, holding it for four, letting it out for four, and pausing for four. Do this a few times, preferably once or twice a day, or if you're feeling anxious.

2. PMR helps relieve physical tension brought on by stress by tensing and relaxing various muscle groups. Before bed, it's very helpful for soothing the body.
    - Tense your muscles for a few seconds at your feet, then let them relax. Breathe deeply as you work your way up through the muscles in your legs, belly, chest, arms, and face.

3. Gratitude Journaling: By thinking back on your good experiences, even the little ones, you may change your viewpoint and reduce stress. According to studies, cultivating thankfulness might enhance mental health and lower inflammation.
    - Write down three things, no matter how minor, for which you are thankful every night. This practice encourages serenity and helps refocus your attention on the positive.

4. Physical Activity: Exercise produces endorphins, which are stress-relieving natural mood boosters. People with autoimmune diseases benefit greatly from physical exercise since it also lowers inflammatory indicators in the body.

- Several times a week, try to get in at least 20 to 30 minutes of moderate exercise, such as yoga, swimming, or walking. The finest activities for maintaining a habit without overexerting yourself are those that are fun and easy on your body.

5. Mindfulness Meditation: Meditation helps you become more emotionally resilient and less stressed by teaching you to notice your thoughts objectively. It has been shown that mindfulness improves general immune function and lowers inflammatory markers.

- Begin by concentrating on your breathing and letting go of distracting ideas for only five minutes each day. If you've never meditated before, guided applications like Calm or Headspace may help you get started.

Relaxation Techniques for Long-Term Relief

Maintaining long-term well-being requires regular relaxation, so it's not simply a one-time thing. By strengthening your mind-gut connection and lowering stress levels, developing a regular relaxation program may help you better control inflammation. Here are some strategies for developing a regular relaxing routine:

1. Establish a Regular Bedtime: Since sleep deprivation may elicit stress and immunological reactions, getting enough sleep is essential for controlling inflammation. Establish a regular nighttime routine to help you get the 7-8 hours of healthy sleep you need. Before going to bed, you may tell your body it's time to relax by reading, stretching gently, or practicing meditation.
2. Create a Relaxation Space at Home: Setting aside a comfortable area for rest will help you detach. Having a place for relaxation, whether it be to read, meditate, or just take deep breaths, serves as a reminder to routinely take time for oneself.
3. Reduce Alcohol and Caffeine: Alcohol and caffeine both raise stress hormones, interfere with sleep, and worsen inflammation. These may be avoided or reduced to assist calm and regulate mood.
4. Connect with Nature: Studies have shown that being outside improves mood, lowers blood pressure, and reduces stress. Short strolls in a local park might provide a soothing, rejuvenating experience that lowers inflammation. Every day, try to spend a few minutes outdoors taking in the sights, sounds, and scents of the environment.
5. Think about Mindful activities: Painting, knitting, or gardening are examples of activities that might help you achieve a flow state, in which you lose yourself entirely in the task at hand. This concentrated mental state is great for lowering stress and promoting mental health.

Selecting the Proper Kind of Exercise

Not all workout is the same when it comes to autoimmune diseases or inflammation. Even while exercise typically improves circulation and lowers inflammation, it's crucial to choose forms of exercise that won't put your body under undue stress or trigger flare-ups. Striking a balance is crucial since too little exercise may make your body stiff and more prone to inflammation, while too much or the incorrect kind of activity can overburden the body and exacerbate symptoms.

Considerations for Selecting Exercises:

1. Low Impact over High Impact: People with autoimmune diseases may experience inflammation and joint stress from high-impact activities like jogging, jumping, and high-intensity interval training (HIIT). Choose low-impact choices instead, since they are less taxing on the body and yet provide great health advantages.

2. Moderation is Key: Try to keep your pace reasonable so you can remain active without becoming tired. Intense exercise or pushing too hard may cause stress hormones to be released, which in some situations can make inflammation worse.

3. Pay Attention to Your Body: Your body will often let you know when it needs to relax or when an activity is too strenuous. Take note of how you feel during and after exercise. Think about changing or substituting milder activities if they cause discomfort or exhaustion.

4. Difference for Whole-Body Wellbeing: Include a variety of exercises for endurance, flexibility, and strength. Exercises for flexibility increase range of motion, strength training protects joints, and cardiovascular health is supported by endurance activities.

Advantages of Low-Impact Activities like Swimming and Yoga

Since low-impact activities are often kinder on the joints while still promoting general health and fitness, they are especially advantageous for those with autoimmune or inflammatory conditions. These activities are perfect for increasing strength, flexibility, and energy levels since they let you keep an active lifestyle without making symptoms worse.

1. Yoga: Yoga helps to improve muscular tone, reduce tension, and promote flexibility by combining exercise with deep breathing and relaxation. Numerous yoga positions improve joint health and reduce stiffness by gradually strengthening and stretching the body. Additionally, yoga promotes attentive movement, which may assist you in being more aware of the requirements and limitations of your body.

- Best Practices: Begin with milder forms of yoga, such as restorative, yin, or hatha. These methods have an emphasis on deep stretches and gradual motions, which are less prone to result in strain. You may enhance your mental health and lower inflammation by doing yoga a few times a week.

2. Swimming: Swimming is a low-impact, full-body exercise that is gentle on the joints. Your body weight is supported by water buoyancy, which eases joint strain and increases your range of motion. Without the startling effect of other types of exercise, swimming may increase flexibility, strengthen muscles, and improve cardiovascular health.

- Best Practices: Start with water aerobics or easy laps if you're new to swimming. Numerous community pools provide sessions for all levels of fitness, including ones tailored to those with inflammatory diseases like arthritis.

3. Walking: Walking is one of the easiest and most accessible types of exercise and is very beneficial for heart health and inflammation reduction. Comfortable walking improves blood flow, lowers stress levels, and preserves joint mobility.

- Best Practices: Try to walk for 20 to 30 minutes every day, or divide that time into shorter walks. Connecting with nature while walking outside has the extra advantage of lowering stress and elevating mood

4. Tai Chi: Tai Chi is a traditional Chinese exercise that combines deep breathing with gentle, flowing motions. Often referred to as "meditation in motion," it is well-known for lowering stress, enhancing equilibrium, and promoting joint health. Because it increases strength and flexibility without putting excessive pressure on the body, tai chi is especially helpful for those with inflammation.

- Best Practices: Although tai chi is usually taught in classrooms, you may learn the fundamentals via a variety of online videos. Stretching, balance, and relaxation may all be significantly improved by practicing for 10 to 20 minutes a few times a week.

Exercise in a Lifestyle That Reduces Inflammation

Beyond improving your physical condition, including exercise into your lifestyle has other advantages. Exercise lowers stress hormones, improves mental health, and helps control immunological responses in those with inflammatory and autoimmune diseases. But in order to get these advantages, moderation and consistency are essential. Here's how to include exercise into your anti-inflammatory regimen in a way that is both sustainable and efficient:

- Develop Routine Slowly: Start out gently and put more emphasis on consistency than intensity if you're new to regular exercise. As you gain comfort, gradually increase the length and frequency of your exercises. This method lowers the chance of inflammatory flare-ups and helps your body adapt without overtaxing it.
- Pay Attention to Balance and Flexibility: Exercises for balance and flexibility increase joint mobility and may help avoid accidents. Stretching or yoga practices on a regular basis may assist ease stiffness and improve the comfort of daily motions. Before and after exercise, even basic stretches may have a significant impact on how your body feels.
- Exercise is a useful tool for reducing stress: By generating endorphins, or "feel-good" chemicals that elevate mood and encourage relaxation, physical exercise naturally lowers stress. These advantages are increased when exercise is combined with mindfulness exercises like yoga or tai chi, which also help to quiet the mind and lower stress chemicals that cause inflammation.
- Give Rest and Recuperation Priority: Days of rest are crucial for recovery and avoiding burnout. It takes time for your immune system, muscles, and joints to heal. Fatigue and increased inflammation might result from over exercising. Give yourself permission to take pauses when necessary and pay attention to your body. On rest days, you may take long walks, meditate, or do some light stretching.
- Be Aware of Nutrition and Hydration: Proper diet and hydration are critical for managing inflammation and recovering after exercise. Stay hydrated by drinking plenty of water, and particularly after working out, feed your body nutrients that reduce inflammation. Inflammation is decreased and muscle regeneration is supported by protein, healthy fats, and fruits and vegetables high in antioxidants.
- Celebrate Your Progress and Set Realistic Goals: Even modest fitness accomplishments may serve as strong motivators. Exercise may be made more pleasurable and satisfying by setting small, attainable

objectives, such as learning a new yoga posture or walking a little further each week. Maintaining your commitment to exercise is made simpler by keeping track of your progress and acknowledging each accomplishment.

- Ask for Help When Needed: Structure and incentive may be obtained by finding an accountability partner, enrolling in a group class, or working with a trainer. A specialist may provide advice on safe workouts and develop a customized plan that meets your requirements, particularly if they are knowledgeable with autoimmune or inflammatory diseases.

When done with awareness, exercise may be a very effective ally in reducing inflammation and autoimmune symptoms. You may design an exercise program that is good for your body and mind by selecting fun, low-impact activities that promote cardiovascular fitness and joint health. An anti-inflammatory lifestyle must include regular, moderate physical exercise since it has been shown to lower inflammation, increase energy, and improve quality of life.

Keep in mind that the objective is to support your body in gentle, regular ways that encourage healing and well-being, not to drive it to its limits. Exercise may be tailored to your individual requirements, whether it's a brisk stroll, a yoga class, or a leisurely swim, paving the way for a long-term journey toward resilience and health.

PERSONAL NOTES

You may record your flare up moments and those happy moments that you feel so energetic in the following pages.

Printed in Dunstable, United Kingdom

65105335R00141